ᵖᵉ

B LANCE
OUR *life*

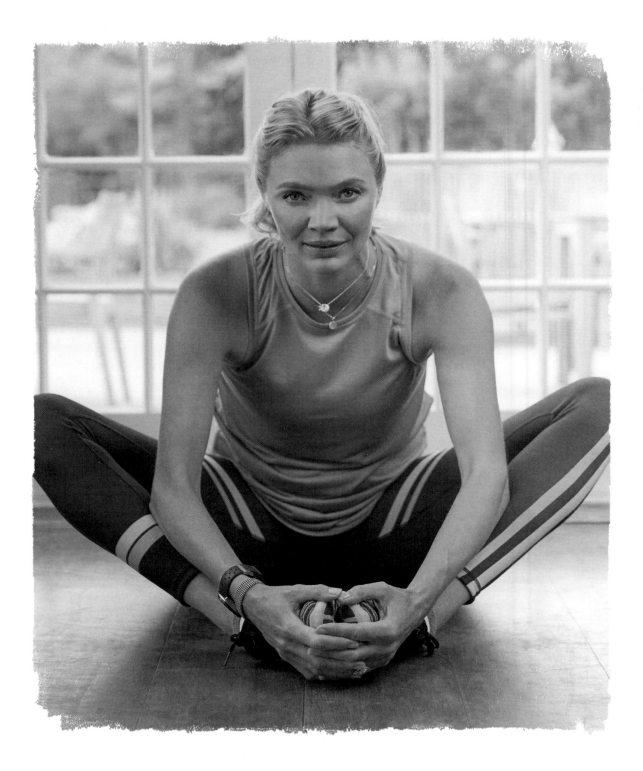

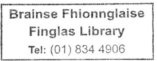
BALANCE
YOUR *life*

a 6-week eating and exercise plan for a calmer, healthier you

AMÉLIE KHELLAF-GOVETT
& JODIE KIDD

CONTENTS

PHASE *ONE*

18

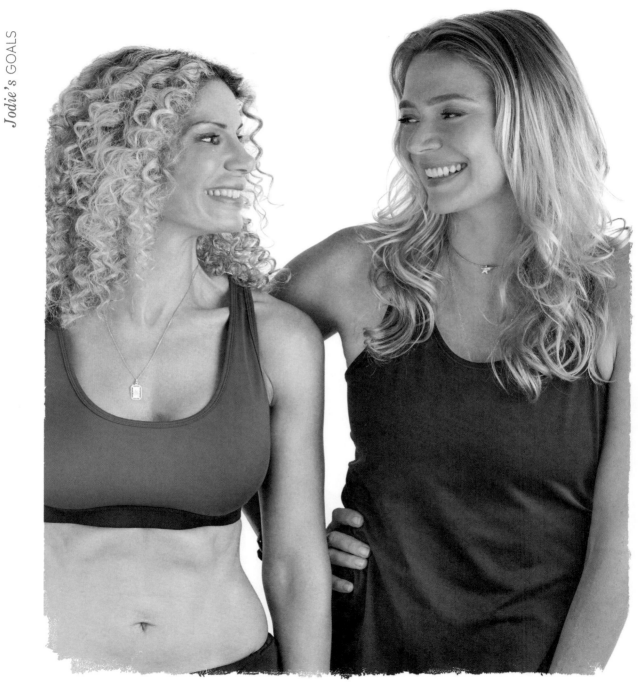

Jodie's GOALS

Over the past few years I've made a lot of big changes to my life. I made it my goal to slow down and spend a bit more time focusing on what's important. These days, in addition to many other things, I run a pub in West Sussex. That role, combined with taking part – and coming runner-up – in Celebrity Masterchef in 2014 furthered my interest in food.

Making changes

When I was modelling I saw food as fuel, but now, working with chefs and growing more aware of the importance of what we put into our bodies, I've really begun to explore the benefits and dangers of the foods we eat, as well as my eating habits. My attitude towards food has changed and I've begun to see its health-giving potential, but I didn't really know where to begin with making, and therefore benefiting from, these changes in my everyday life. We're bombarded with so many mixed messages about what's good for us, and what's not, that making healthy choices can feel like a minefield.

A big birthday this year also made me sit up and take notice of my body in ways I never had before. I've been on a mission to boost my energy and mental clarity, and to ease some of the anxiety I often feel. That is what's made me embark on Amélie's programme. I love Amélie's promise of achieving the balance so many of us need in our lives.

Find your balance

We live in a time where we constantly feel pressure to be perfect and to get it right. But it's all about having a lifestyle that you make work for you, not that you have to conform to. Amélie's programme is realistic for a 40-year-old mum, or any woman for that matter. She believes you don't have to beat yourself up for being a real person. If you give in to temptation one day, you just know you need to do a little bit better the next day. The programme isn't off-puting and you can enjoy the process – and your life – while you're at it.

I hope you find as much success with Amélie's programme as I have. Just remember, the most important things are to be kind to yourself and find your natural balance.

Amélie's PROMISE

As a personal trainer I want to help you to lose weight and feel better in yourself without starving you or making you feel terribly frustrated.

If I could choose just one mission in life it would be to help people make peace with food and exercise, and encourage them to realize that looking after yourself is not just a matter of aesthetics. A healthy body gives you a healthy mind, and vice versa; it's a two-way relationship. However, when it comes to your nutrition and fitness, as an adult, you need to exercise some discipline and control over your day-to-day choices.

Eat right

The eating plan I've devised minimizes sugar intake in all its forms, and that means refined sugar and carbohydrates. Eating sugar will not only make you fat, but it will also make you crave even more sugar. My method shows you how to prepare meals and generally eat foods that score low on the Glycaemic Index (GI). Foods that score high on this index, such as white bread and pasta, contain carbohydrates that cause blood-sugar levels to shoot up at a very high rate in your system. When this happens, you get hungry, you get anxious, you want more sugar, and – in time – you store all the unnecessary energy generated by the sugar as fat and you gain weight. That's without even talking about diabetes, high cholesterol, and the other myriad health problems that come with prolonged high blood-sugar levels. For all these reasons, it is important to avoid eating high-GI foods. Eating low-GI foods, which feature in my plan, minimizes any rise in blood-sugar levels, and even stops them going up.

However, if it were as easy as explaining the science and simply avoiding high-GI foods, few people in our society would have issues with weight gain due to consuming too much sugar. Yet just a glance around will tell you this is not the case. This is because, as a species, we are hard-wired to crave sugar in all its forms. Babies will usually take something sweet over something bitter or tangy, as sugar is a key fuel for their growing brains.

More insidiously, in our society, sugar is everywhere. As children, we're given sweet treats as a reward. This continues into adulthood, when the most easily available foods are often high in sugar. The reality is that sugar in all its forms is like an addictive – yet legal – drug. Many processed foods – even most savoury ready-meals – actually contain refined sugar, so my plan completely cuts them out. Conversely, cooking with low-GI foods will help you lose the sugar habit and restore your enjoyment of eating real food. Ultimately, you'll find that you reach the point where tasting something very sweet actually burns your mouth.

A balanced approach

The key is to bring your brain with you on your journey. As the name of the book implies, my method promotes a balanced way of eating, where you can have all sorts of foods and enjoy delicious meals. The method doesn't ban any food apart from processed food. It helps you make the right choices and understand that everything is linked: your body reacts to everything you put into it, and so does your mind. And you can still have a little bit of most things, but not too often.

The plan is flexible, of course, but bear in mind that everything you put into your mouth will have an impact on its outcome. If you want this six-week plan to work for you, you need to be very mindful of what you eat from the start. Make sure your meals are balanced, that you eat enough vegetables and protein, that all your carbohydrates are wholegrain, and that you're

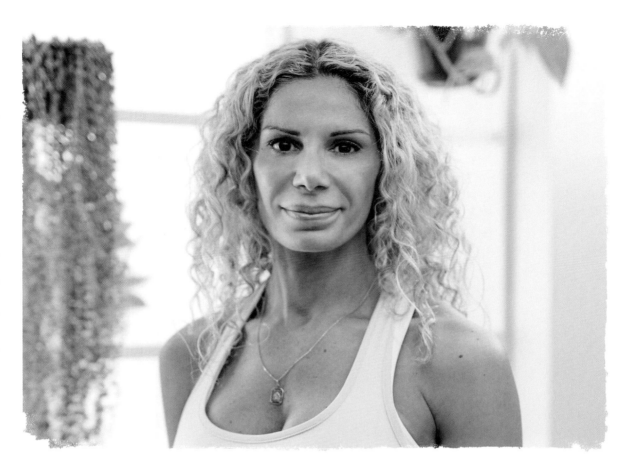

cooking these properly. For example, even wholegrain pasta should be served al dente so it doesn't cause a spike in your blood-sugar levels, while fruit should not be eaten too ripe.

Find your passion

As for exercise, it's okay not to be in the mood every day to "kill it" while working out. We are not machines, we are all different ages, and many of us have busy lives. But you should try to be as active as you can. After the six weeks are over, I urge you to go and find something that you really enjoy doing. Perhaps on one day do a dance class, on another day do some strength training, and another day take a bike ride with the kids. Stay active and always bear in mind that being sedentary and static

will work against you 100 per cent. The little things make a difference: get off the bus one stop early; ban the lift and always take the stairs; get out and get fresh air at lunchtime. Just move. Be active – not hyperactive – and feel free to experiment.

The book is a blueprint, intended to give you an appetite for exercise of whatever kind suits you best. I am a fitness professional, but even I've had to experiment with different things because I get bored. I needed to find something I absolutely loved doing that would get me out of bed. Always use your head as well as your body. Have a good chat with yourself, explore lots of ways to get yourself (and keep yourself) moving, and find out what really works for you.

A word on...

My plan has a carefully designed structure involving nutrition and fitness to help you develop a healthy mind–body balance. I want to help you lose weight and feel better in yourself, but I never forget that each of us is unique, with our own metabolism, life story, and aspirations.

For this reason, I am offering twelve tips to help you better understand how the plan will work for you. Read them through before you begin, and think about how they relate to your story. In which areas do you feel confident? Where do you feel you need extra support? Refer to these tips from time to time to help you keep your focus and stick to the plan.

1 Success

The way you measure success is highly personal. Some people like weigh-ins (only once a week, please) or taking measurements (only every two weeks). Some like visual cues, so a fortnightly before-and-after photo will suit them better. For others, it's about how they feel in their skin and clothes, so a particular item of clothing – a tight pair of jeans, for example – is the perfect benchmark.

2 Kindness

Be kind to yourself. Embarking on a healthier journey is not a punishment for having a ful -on life. Being busy can easily lead to us making the wrong choices for our bodies and minds. Now is the time to step back, take a deep breath, and think about how the plan is going to work for you, to make your body and mind stronger and healthier, and to help alleviate stress.

3 Satisfaction

Our brains are wired to embrace pleasure and fight deprivation, so it's paramount that the meals you make are always satisfying and enjoyable. To help with this, use herbs and spices to jazz up your food. Enjoying a meal that makes you happy is an extra weapon against cravings and snacking.

4 Cravings

These are part of life. Constant y fighting them exhausts your mind and body (there's only so much struggle your system can tolerate). Approach cravings with moderation: it's better in the long run to have a small portion of chips or a few mouthfuls of cake than fight the craving and end up binge ng later. As long as this isn't a daily occurrence, it won't hinder your progress.

5 *Using your head*

Embarking on a nutritional overhaul hinges on 50 per cent motivation, 30 per cent food choices, and 20 per cent logistics (shopping, cooking, and so on). With this in mind, using your head at all times is pivotal to success. Motivation comes from within and on days that you are not feeling it, you can talk yourself back into it. Remember, you've got this.

6 *"But I didn't eat all day!"*

Sometimes this statement is true and sometimes it's not accurate at all. Just because you didn't have a full meal, or didn't sit down to have food, doesn't mean you didn't eat. Picking is eating. If you find yourself finishing your kid's food at every meal, that is also eating. So make sure there's the right amount, just for them.

7 *Eating out*

Socializing and travelling are part of life. There is no need to choose the most boring dish; take your time to scan a menu and think about what will work. The perfect combination is a starter and a main course, but if you fancy a dessert, drop the starter. Choose the least sugary dessert. Your goal is to minimize sugar consumption (white carbs) and processed foods.

8 *Bed*

Your bed is for two things: sleep and sex. Try not to take your laptop, tablet, phone, or any other electronic device into the bedroom. The pre-sleep stimulation caused by looking at a screen is catastrophic for your sleep quality, and this has repercussions for every aspect of your health. If you use your phone to wake up in the morning, invest in an alarm clock instead.

9 *Concentrating while training*

Think about the movements you are performing and focus on the muscles that you are working and engaging. It's more "mind with matter" than "mind over matter". Staying in the moment while training makes your body work harder and bring results quicker. Honest training = honest results.

10 *"Burning off" excess*

You can't out-train a bad diet. It's a fact and not much can be done about it. Changing the way you look starts with putting some thought into what's on your plate. Training is designed to enhance the results of better nutrition.

11 *Delayed onset muscle soreness (DOMS)*

This is the pain you feel the day after working out. It's not pleasant. In a way it is quite gratifying, however, because it is tangible proof that your body has put in the work. For some people the pain is more intense two days after a session. No need to panic, it will subside.

12 *Rest days*

Muscles are – surprisingly – built when you are resting and not when you are training. It's important to stick to the rest-day pattern given for each phase.

Amélie's
FOOD PHILOSOPHY

The whole programme covered in this book lasts for six weeks and is broken down into three 2-week eating plans: "Declutter", "Fight", and "Preserve". The goal is to rebalance your nutrition and get you to a point where you are comfortable and in control when it comes to your food choices. The idea is that, at the end of six weeks, you will have learned to enjoy a new way of eating that balances pleasure and discipline.

1 In the morning, **brush your teeth** before drinking or eating anything. This will get rid of bacteria that have built up overnight and protect your teeth from acidity.

2 **Drink warm cinnamon and lemon** before anything else. Let the hot water tap run for about 20 seconds while you rinse a lemon and cut it in half (you will only use half a lemon in the drink). Squeeze the lemon half into a mug, drop the squeezed-out lemon half in too, cover with the warm tap water, then add a pinch of ground cinnamon.

Sip it slowly – you can use a straw (preferably paper) to protect your teeth – as you're getting ready for the day.

3 **Drink 1.5–2 litres (2¾–3½ pints) of water every day.** Always have a bottle nearby, as you will use it to reduce snacking: every time you feel like snacking, drink up!

4 **Cut out alcohol.** Alcohol is pure sugar, and sugar gets stored around the waist and hips, which is counterproductive when working towards a flatter stomach. Alcohol also slows down your

metabolism: the opposite of what we are trying to achieve with this programme. It's also important to remember that alcohol is a depressant and it reduces the chemical signals travelling around the brain.

5 **Eat sitting down**. Whether it's an apple or a full-on meal, sit down to eat it. If it's not worth sitting down for, it's not worth eating.

6 Whatever is not water is food. Get in the habit of **thinking about what you put in your mouth**, not in an obsessive way, but in a conscious educated way. Train your brain to discern the difference between "I am hungry" and "I feel like eating". Chances are, you haven't actually gone hungry in a very long time; our environment, society, and lifestyle have taken over from our ability to recognize true hunger. Whether it's a fake aroma of warm croissants pumped out in the supermarket, or browsing Instagram

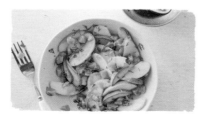 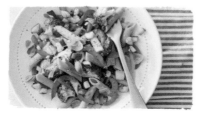 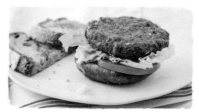

and being hit by dozens of food photos, these are all triggers that trick our brains into thinking we're hungry when, really, we're merely giving in to a reflex. It's very important that you use the first two weeks of the plan to rehabilitate your brain and train yourself to eat only when you're really hungry.

7 Unless you stole it, you should **never feel guilty** about the food you eat. Guilt is a strong negative feeling that will raise your cortisol level, which in turn makes the hunger hormone – ghrelin – go through the roof.

8 **Never shop for groceries when hungry** and always make a detailed list beforehand. I highly recommend online shopping, as there is no scope to browse snack or chocolate aisles, or to be tempted by colourful snack wrappers while queuing. It also allows you to take your time to think about what you're buying and why; for example, with

the aim of making home-cooked meals from scratch three times a week.

9 **Do not buy anything labelled "fat-free" or "sugar-free"** (they tend to contain artificial sweeteners and other unnatural ingredients, all of which are hunger-inducing), or "white" products, such as white pasta, rice, bread, or couscous. These all turn into sugar, which, once digested, turns into fat. This type of fat lodges itself on the stomach and hip areas. We don't want that…

10 Portion control is important and can be exercised in different ways:
- **Use smaller plates**. If your dinner plates are big, you'll eat more. Use a side plate instead and stop eating when you're no longer hungry, rather than when you're full.
- **Never eat from a packet**: always decant your food. It's fine to have chocolate from time to time, but

learn to break off a couple of squares, then put the bar away. Whatever you fancy eating, transfer your portion to a small bowl or plate. It's less lethal than dipping your hand into a bag until it's finished, and is a simple trick that teaches you moderation.

11 Lastly – and this is probably the most important aspect of my method – **balance your nutrition**. Balance is diametrically opposed to the "all or nothing" approach that has sabotaged our metabolisms for decades. It's about making clear, conscious, rational decisions. Had a big dinner? Have light meals the following day. Had a festive weekend with a succession of rich meals washed down with wine? Then next week needs to be about good, healthy foods, and alcohol free. This is the only way to still be able to enjoy everything you like and not ruin your efforts in the process.

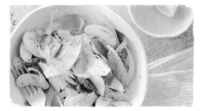
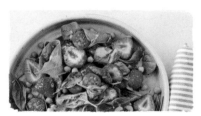
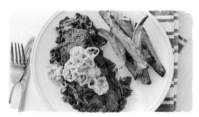

Amélie's EXERCISE PHILOSOPHY

The exercise in this book is broken down into three 2-week exercise plans : "Ignite", "Body training", and "Success". I've devised a training method based on metabolic conditioning, which is a ruthlessly effective way to burn fat while building muscle. It will improve your flexibility, balance, and heart health, and it's also been proven to regulate hunger hormones. Most importantly, it's challenging and fun and will make you feel like you can take on anything the day throws at you.

1 Before you get out of bed, take five seconds to **stretch your entire body**, starfish style.

2 **You will need** a timer and two 2–3kg (4½–6½lb) dumbbells to complete the exercises in the three phases. You may also want an exercise mat. Make sure you have these to hand before starting the programme.

3 When doing most exercises, aim to **have your feet about 50cm (20in) apart**, unless otherwise specified.

4 **Be aware of your "energy benchmark"**: how much energy you have to spend and what you can manage. This will help you adapt the intensity of your effort and prevent you from skipping a training session.

5 **Make sure that your posture is correct** at all times, to avoid injuries and maximize results. Remember the cardinal rules when it comes to posture: shoulders down and back, navel drawing towards your spine, and knees soft and slightly bent.

6 **It's okay to train when you have your period**. Unless you have very painful cramps, it won't impact on your physical performance. Make sure you drink more water than usual to avoid becoming dehydrated.

7 **Take a view on training while you're ill**. If you have congestion and a dry cough, you're good to go. If you have symptoms in your chest or stomach, steer clear. Working out with a fever is a definite no-no. Recuperate and take care of yourself for a few days instead.

8 **Remember to breathe** while working out: never hold your breath. Instead, inhale on the easiest part of the exercise and exhale during the most difficult part. Concentrate on slowing down your breath during the cool-down phase of your exercise routine.

9 **Stay hydrated**. When exercising, keep a water bottle close to your exercise mat and drink from it frequently during the short rest breaks.

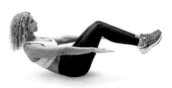
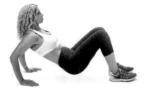

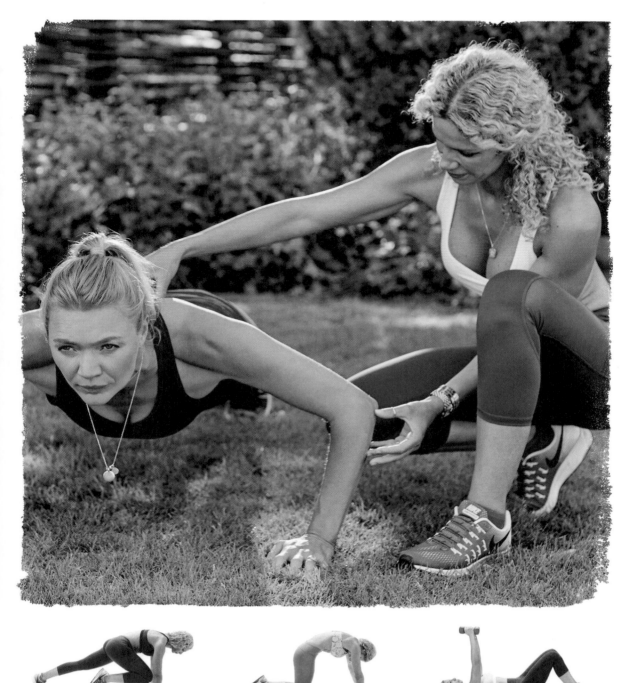

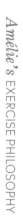

THE PLAN
at a glance

Here we have pulled together all the elements of the Balance Your Life plan to give you an at-a-glance overview of what's involved.

The plan is designed around three two-week phases.

In each two-week phase, the first seven days is repeated in the second week.

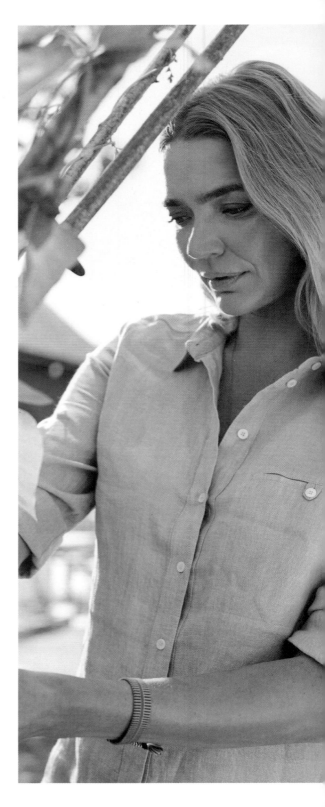

PHASE *ONE*
weeks 1–2

This is a nutrition and exercise plan designed to:

- Rid your body and mind of toxic behaviours
- Kick off the weight-loss process
- Ignite your metabolism

DECLUTTER EATING PLAN

During this stage, you will also take some time to think and makes notes about how you respond to stress or anxiety, and to develop an awareness of your emotional responses to food.

IGNITE EXERCISE PLAN

The Ignite Exercise Plan is a bodyweight-based workout that will help you burn fat and build muscle.

PHASE *TWO*
weeks 3–4

In the second stage the focus shifts, and the nutrition plan and exercises help you:

- Fight stubborn fat
- Achieve muscle definition

FIGHT EATING PLAN

Once a week in this stage you will do a "Fire Fight Day". This involves a screen detox, where you avoid looking at social media or emails from 9pm the night before.

BODY TRAINING EXERCISE PLAN

The Body Training Exercise Plan will continue your muscle-building progress, making you stronger and giving you more muscle definition.

PHASE *THREE*
weeks 5–6

This final stage takes you to the finishing line, and instils lifelong behavioural mechanisms that enable you to:

- Keep boosting the fat-burning process
- Make use of the mental and physical tools you now have, for making the right nutritional choices conducive to weight loss and general wellbeing

PRESERVE EATING PLAN

A unique feature of this stage is the "Sans Day", for which you will select one food from a list of several to give up for the day. This helps with fat loss and also keeps you in control of your diet and food choices.

SUCCESS EXERCISE PLAN

The Success Exercise Plan is designed to continue the work you do in the first four weeks, and take you forward long after Phase Three is over.

PHASE ONE

weeks 1–2

The first two weeks of the programme rid your body and mind of toxic behaviours and kick off the weight-loss process with a nutrition and exercise plan designed to fire up your metabolism. It's broken down into a **DECLUTTER EATING PLAN** and a 30-minute **IGNITE EXERCISE PLAN**.

DECLUTTER
eating plan

This is the meal plan you will follow over the next two weeks. It's designed to cut out sugar. Days 1–6 are laid out for you in detail, but for Day 7 you can choose your favourite meals from the week, or try a new recipe from Jodie. Once you reach the end of Week 1, go back and repeat the plan for Week 2.

Remember to drink a glass of the warm cinnamon and lemon water in the morning before you have anything else (see p12.)

Remember to eat only when you're sitting down, and to drink 1.5–2 liters (2¾–3½ pints) of water every day.

I have given you seven breakfast options (see pp 24–25) to choose from. You don't need to eat a different one each day; you can pick and choose the ones you like and repeat them as many times throughout the two weeks as you like.

You can choose one snack from the options on page 25 to have each afternooon. As with breakfasts, you can choose whichever snack appeals to you most.

Finish your day with a mug of herbal tea such as liquorice, cinnamon, jasmine, or green tea. This will become the signal to your brain that you're done eating for the day.

On Day 7 you can choose to make Jodie's recipes (see pp44–47) instead of repeating recipes from earlier in the week.

You will need a steamer, non-stick frying pan, and kitchen scales to hand.

BREAKFAST
LUNCH
DINNER
BREAKFAST
LUNCH
DINNER
BREAKFAST
LUNCH
DINNER
BREAKFAST
LUNCH
DINNER

Weeks 1–2

DAY 1	DAY 2
Choose from the selection on pages 24–25	Choose from the selection on pages 24–25
Chicken and crudités	Lemon salmon papillote
Turkey with sautéed garlic broccoli	Indian rice

DAY 3	DAY 4
Choose from the selection on pages 24–25	Choose from the selection on pages 24–25
Avocado and salmon tartare	Salade Parisienne
Crudités, burger, and quinoa	Cod á l'Italienne

DAY 5	DAY 6
Choose from the selection on pages 24–25	Choose from the selection on pages 24–25
Salade à la Grecque	Lemony chicken
Salmon with creamed spinach	Penne primavera

DAY 7	
Choose from the selection on pages 24–25	
Choose your favourite lunch recipe from the week, or try one of Jodie's recipes	
Choose your favourite dinner recipe from the week, or try one of Jodie's recipes	

A word on triggers

I strongly recommend that you take some time to think about your food "triggers". Start making notes of your reaction to any form of stress or anxiety, and generally develop an emotional consciousness towards food.

DECLUTTER
weekly shopping list

Here's the basic list of ingredients you'll need for lunch and dinner every day for Days 1–6 of the plan. Breakfasts, snacks, and your Day 7 meals are your choice, so the ingredients and quantities are not included below. Bear in mind that all meats, fish, fruits, and vegetables need to be organic. You will also need to buy extra for Days 7 and 14, when you choose your favourite meal from the week or one of Jodie's recipes to cook, and for desserts. Make sure you have a steamer, non-stick frying pans, and kitchen scales.

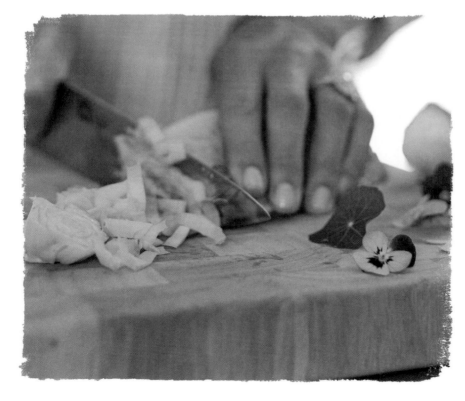

Fruits and vegetables

Apples 2
Granny Smith,
Pink Lady,
or Gala

Avocados 1

Broccoli
200–250g (7–9oz)

Carrots
unlimited, for
crudités

Celery
unlimited, for
crudités

Courgettes 2

Cucumbers
unlimited, for crudités,
plus an extra 100g
(3½oz)

Garlic 1 head

**Green beans, extra
fine** 150g (5½oz)

Herbs
Buy your herbs in
bunches or packs.
You will need:
Basil
Coriander
Dill
Mint
Flat-leaf parsley

Lemons 7

Lettuce 2 handfuls
Romaine and/or your
favourite salad leaves

Red pepper 1

Shallots 2

Spinach
200g (7oz) bag,
or as much as
you want

Sweet potato
150g (5½oz)

Tomatoes, cherry
unlimited, for crudités
plus 100g (3½oz)

Tomatoes, regular
100g (3½oz) for
chopping

Meat, fish, and eggs

Beef, minced (lean)
80g (3oz)

**Chicken breast meat,
cooked, free-range**
180g (6¼oz)

**Chicken breasts,
raw, free-range** 2
100g (3½oz) each

Cod 150g (5½oz)

Salmon fillets, wild
3 fillets, 200g (7oz) each

**Turkey, cooked
free-range**
3 slices

**Turkey breast,
raw, free-range**
100g (3½oz)

Dairy and non-dairy alternatives

**Cream cheese, full-fat,
or non-dairy
alternative**
2 tbsp

Crème fraîche, half-fat
90g (3¼oz)

Feta cheese
30g (1oz)

Store cupboard

Here is a list of the
supplies you will need to
have to hand. Make sure
you keep stocked up on
these so you don't run
out as you work your way
through the phases

Bread, wholemeal

Cinnamon, ground

Cumin, ground

Curry powder

Dark agave syrup

**Extra virgin olive oil
spray**

**Extra virgin organic
olive oil**

Greaseproof paper

Mustard, Dijon

**Pasta, wholegrain
penne**

Quinoa

Rice, brown

**Soy sauce,
reduced salt**

Vinegar, balsamic

Beverage

Herbal tea
Any of your choice

**Water, sparkling
or still**
You can choose either,
as long as every day you
drink 1.5–2 litres (2¾–
3½ pints)

Breakfasts, snacks, and
herbal teas are all your
choice. Look through the
recipes (pp26–41), decide
what you'd like to eat, and
then shop accordingly.

BREAKFASTS *and* SNACKS

For the first two weeks, eat one of these breakfasts each morning. It doesn't matter if you have the same one several times and don't try the others – they are all good for you. Portions are for one person. If you are hungry after lunch, you can have one of the snacks, opposite, in the afternoon.

Breakfast options

Option 1

WHOLEMEAL BREAD
2 slices with a thin layer of butter

+

1 BOILED EGG
(boiled to your liking)

+

1 CLEMENTINE

Option 2

OVERNIGHT OATS
The night before serving, half-fill a small bowl or a mug with rolled oats and just cover with water. Sweeten with 1 tsp agave syrup, if you like. Stir, cover, and refrigerate overnight.

+

2 SLICES COOKED FREE-RANGE TURKEY

+

1 KIWI FRUIT

Option 3

WHOLEMEAL BREAD
2 slices with a thin layer of peanut butter

+

1 BOILED EGG
(boiled to your liking)

+

BLUEBERRIES
½ small bowl, or ½ mug

Snack options
Choose any one of these snacks to eat in the afternoon to bridge the gap between lunch and dinner.

Option 1

1 APPLE

Option 2

FULL-FAT YOGURT
½ small bowl, or ½ mug, plain yogurt, sweetened with 1 tsp agave syrup

Option 3

GREEN GRAPES
1 small bowl or mug

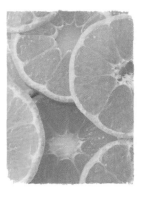
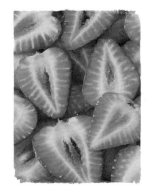
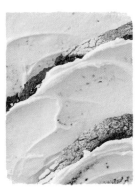
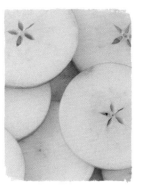

Option 4

WHOLEMEAL BREAD
2 slices with a thin layer of butter

+

FULL-FAT YOGURT
½ small bowl, or ½ mug, plain yogurt, sweetened with 1 tsp agave syrup

+

5 ALMONDS
(mixed with the yogurt, if you like)

Option 5

OVERNIGHT OATS
(see Option 2)

+

2 SLICES COOKED FREE-RANGE CHICKEN

+

1 CLEMENTINE

Option 6

AVOCADO TOAST
2 slices wholegrain bread with ½ avocado, mashed

+

YOGURT
½ small bowl, or ½ mug, full-fat plain yogurt, sweetened with 1 tsp agave syrup

+

STRAWBERRIES
½ small bowl, or ½ mug

Option 7

WHOLEMEAL BREAD
2 slices with a thin layer of cream cheese, or non-dairy alternative

+

2-EGG OMELETTE
Cover a small frying pan with extra virgin olive oil spray and place over a medium heat. Lightly beat 2 eggs in a small bowl, adding a small handful of chopped soft herbs, if you wish. Pour the eggs into the pan and cook to your liking.

+

1 APPLE

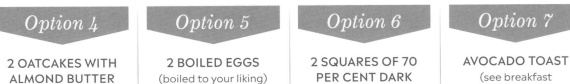

Option 4

2 OATCAKES WITH ALMOND BUTTER

Option 5

2 BOILED EGGS
(boiled to your liking)

Option 6

2 SQUARES OF 70 PER CENT DARK CHOCOLATE WITH A CUP OF HERBAL TEA

Option 7

AVOCADO TOAST
(see breakfast Option 6)

DAY 1

Breakfast

Choose from the selection on pages 24–25

Choose from the selection on pages 24–25

Lunch

CHICKEN AND CRUDITÉS

SERVES 1

100g (3½oz) skinless, boneless free-range chicken breast

salt and pepper

100g (3½oz) brown rice

raw vegetables (as many as you want): carrots, cucumber, celery, chopped into batons, and cherry tomatoes, halved

1 tbsp full-fat cream cheese, or non-dairy alternative

1 Preheat the oven to 200°C (400°F/Gas 6). Line a baking sheet with greaseproof paper.

2 Cook the chicken on the prepared baking sheet for 25–30 minutes, or until it is no longer pink on the inside when sliced. Season with salt and pepper, to taste.

3 Meanwhile, cook the rice according to the packet instructions.

4 Serve the chicken and rice with the raw vegetables and cream cheese.

Dessert

5 level tbsp soya yogurt

Snack

Choose a snack from the list on page 25
(optional, only if you're hungry)

Choose a snack from the list on page 25 (optional, only if you're hungry)

Dinner

TURKEY WITH SAUTÉED GARLIC BROCCOLI

SERVES 1

100g (3½oz) free-range turkey breast

salt and pepper

small bowl of broccoli florets

extra virgin olive oil spray

2 garlic cloves, finely chopped

1 Preheat the oven to 200°C (400°F/Gas 6). Line a baking sheet with greaseproof paper.

2 Cook the turkey on the prepared baking sheet for 20–25 minutes, or until it is no longer pink on the inside when sliced. Season with salt and pepper, to taste, and set aside.

3 Steam the broccoli for about 5 minutes. (Make sure it doesn't become too soft, because overcooked vegetables lose their nutrients.)

4 Spray 2 squirts of extra virgin olive oil spray into a frying pan, place over a very low heat, and add the garlic. When the garlic is soft and aromatic, add the broccoli, increase the heat to medium, and sauté for about 3 minutes. Serve warm with the cooked turkey.

Dessert

small mug of strawberries
2 squares 70 per cent cocoa solids chocolate

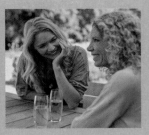

Jodie & Amélie

66 *Amélie*

What are your goals food-wise
during the plan?

Jodie

I'm hoping to get more energy and
head space. I want to be kinder to
my body and look after myself. I'd like
to change my mindset and relationship
with food and reset my habits. **99**

66 *Amélie*

What is your current relationship
and mindset with food?

Jodie

Since opening the pub I've begun to look at
food differently. When I was modelling I saw
food as fuel. As I've got older I've tried to be
more mindful about what I eat, but it's hard
to keep it up all of the time when you're
a busy working mum. **99**

I've found that the exercises are making me feel stronger, more energized, and giving me better mental clarity. It makes me feel like I can get on with my day and fix anything.

- Jodie

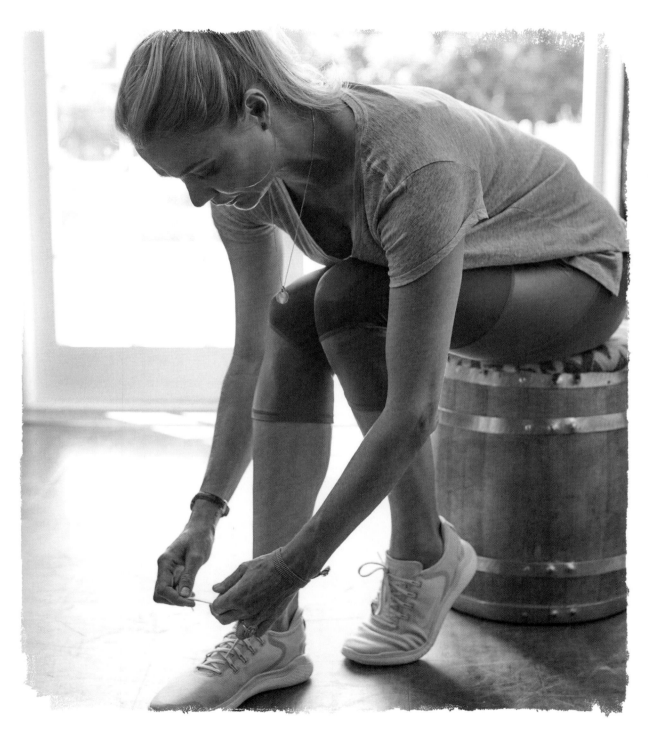

DAY 2

Breakfast

Choose from the selection on pages 24–25

Lunch

LEMON SALMON PAPILLOTE

SERVES 1

1 wild salmon fillet, about 200g (7oz)

1 lemon slice

leaves from 2 sprigs of coriander, chopped

salt and pepper

150g (5oz) extra-fine green beans

1 slice wholemeal bread

1 Preheat the oven to 200°C (400°F/Gas 6).

2 Make a little parcel with greaseproof paper. Place the salmon fillet in it and top with a slice of lemon. Sprinkle with chopped coriander and season with salt and pepper. Fold the paper to seal the seams and cook in the oven for 10–12 minutes.

3 Meanwhile, steam the green beans for 3–5 minutes, or until firm but tender.

4 Remove the salmon from the papillote and serve with the beans and wholemeal bread.

Dessert

1 apple

Snack

Choose a snack from the list on page 25 (optional, only if you're hungry)

Dinner

INDIAN RICE

SERVES 1

100g (3½oz) skinless, boneless free-range chicken breast

salt and pepper

1 tsp olive oil

1 shallot, finely chopped

100g (3½oz) brown rice

1 tsp curry powder

1 Preheat the oven to 200°C (400°F/Gas 6). Line a baking sheet with greaseproof paper.

2 Cook the chicken on the prepared baking sheet for 25–30 minutes, or until it is no longer pink on the inside when sliced. Season with salt and pepper, to taste.

3 Warm the oil in a saucepan over a low heat. Add the shallot and rice. Stir, then leave to cook for 3–4 minutes. Add 200ml (7fl oz) of water. Stir in the curry powder and leave to cook for about 15 minutes.

4 Serve the rice with the chicken.

Dessert

½ bowl full-fat plain yogurt drizzled with 1 tsp agave syrup

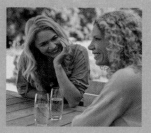

Jodie & Amélie

" *Amélie*

What challenges do you anticipate while doing the 6-week plan?

Jodie

I travel a lot and it's not always easy to find healthy options or the time and space to work out. Running the pub also means there is a lot of temptation. Sometimes it can be hard to resist a glass of wine or two. **"**

" *Amélie*

It can be hard to fit a strict diet into real life. Things are going to come up, but you can't live in isolation with rules. Discipline is good to have, but rigidity is not.

Jodie

That's what I liked about this plan. Your philosophy is about balance. You don't need to panic if you indulge and have dessert when you're out to dinner with friends, you just do a few more minutes of exercise, or eat a little less, the next day. **"**

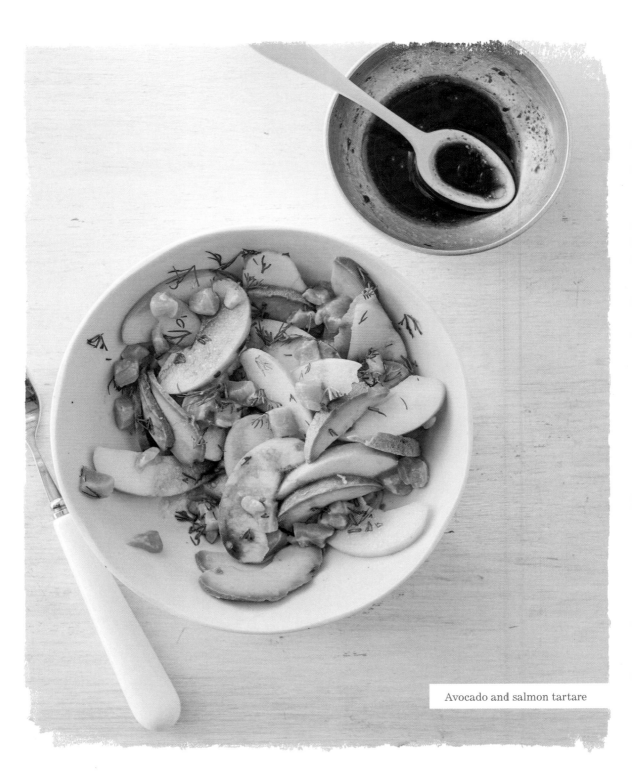

Avocado and salmon tartare

DAY 3

Breakfast

Choose from the selection on pages 24–25

Lunch

AVOCADO AND SALMON TARTARE

SERVES 1

For the tartare

1 skinless, boneless wild salmon fillet*, about 200g (7oz)

juice of 1 lemon

1 tart eating apple (such as Granny Smith)

½ avocado

small handful of dill, chopped

For the dressing

1 tsp extra virgin olive oil

1 tsp balsamic vinegar

1 tsp reduced salt soy sauce

1 Finely chop the salmon, place in a small bowl, and cover with half the lemon juice.

2 Peel and slice the apple and avocado half and place in a separate small bowl. Cover with the remaining lemon juice.

3 Make the dressing by whisking all the ingredients in another bowl, cup, or jar, until thoroughly mixed.

4 In a serving bowl, stir together the salmon, apple, and avocado. Cover with the dressing, sprinkle with the dill, and serve.

Dessert

5 level tbsp full-fat plain yogurt with natural flavouring

*Before eating raw salmon, ensure it has been frozen according to EFSA guidelines.

Snack

Choose a snack from the list on page 25
(optional, only if you're hungry)

Dinner

CRUDITÉS, BURGER, AND QUINOA

SERVES 1

For the burger and quinoa

100g (3½oz) quinoa

80g (2¾oz) lean minced beef

small handful of chopped coriander leaves

small handful of chopped mint leaves

½ tsp ground cumin

For the crudités

raw vegetables (as many as you want): carrots, cucumber, celery, chopped into batons, and cherry tomatoes, halved

1 tbsp full-fat cream cheese, or non-dairy alternative

1 Cook the quinoa according to the packet instructions.

2 In a bowl, mix the beef with the herbs and cumin. Wet your hands slightly, then form the mixture into a patty.

3 Place a non-stick frying pan over a medium heat. Add the patty to the pan and cook for 5 minutes a side, turning once, or until cooked to your liking. First serve the crudités with the cream cheese for dipping, and then the burger with the quinoa.

Dessert

BAKED CINNAMON APPLE

1 apple

1 tsp ground cinnamon

Preheat the oven to 180°C (350°F/Gas 4). Score the apple around its equator, then core it. Sprinkle with the cinnamon, making sure to get some into the hole left by the core. Bake for 20 minutes, or until tender.

DAY 4

Breakfast

Choose from the selection on pages 24–25

Lunch

SALADE PARISIENNE

SERVES 1

For the salad

2 handfuls of your favourite green salad leaves

100g (3½oz) tomatoes, chopped

150g (5½oz) cooked brown rice

80g (2¾oz) skinless, boneless free range chicken breast, cooked and chopped

For the dressing

1 tsp extra virgin olive oil

juice of ½ lemon, or to taste

½ shallot, very finely chopped

small handful of flat-leaf parsley leaves, chopped

½ tsp Dijon mustard, or to taste

salt and pepper

1 Mix the green salad leaves, tomatoes, rice, and chicken together in a serving bowl.

2 Now, in a small bowl or cup, whisk together all the ingredients for the dressing until thoroughly mixed. Taste and adjust the levels of lemon juice or mustard.

3 Drizzle the salad with the dressing and toss gently to coat.

Dessert

1 apple

Snack

Choose a snack from the list on page 25 (optional, only if you're hungry)

Dinner

COD À L'ITALIENNE

SERVES 1

2 tomatoes, sliced

150g (5½oz) cod fillet

60g (2oz) half-fat crème fraîche

2 shallots, very finely chopped

juice of ½ lemon, or to taste

1 tsp Dijon mustard, or to taste

salt and pepper

150g (5½oz) sweet potato, peeled and cut into chunks

1 Preheat the oven to 200°C (400°F/Gas 6). Spread the slices from one of the tomatoes on the bottom of an ovenproof dish and place the cod on top.

2 In a bowl, mix together the crème fraîche, shallots, lemon juice, and mustard, and season with salt and pepper. Adjust the seasoning and mustard, to taste.

3 Cover the cod with the mixture, then set the remaining slices of tomato on top. Bake for 20 minutes, or until the fish is opaque all the way through.

4 Meanwhile, steam the sweet potato chunks for 20 minutes. Serve them with the cod.

Dessert

1 apple

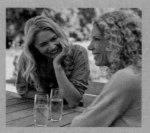

Jodie & Amélie

 Amélie
What would you say is your
worst habit around food?

Jodie
I love cheese with a glass of wine and was
starting to indulge myself more than necessary.
It became a habit, but there are things you
should eat for pleasure on occasion, rather
than just out of habit. "

Amélie
And how are you feeling now
after a few days?

Jodie
You feel really good when you don't drink!
The extra energy I've gained from not
drinking has made me not miss that
evening glass of wine. I know I'll feel so
much better if I don't indulge. "

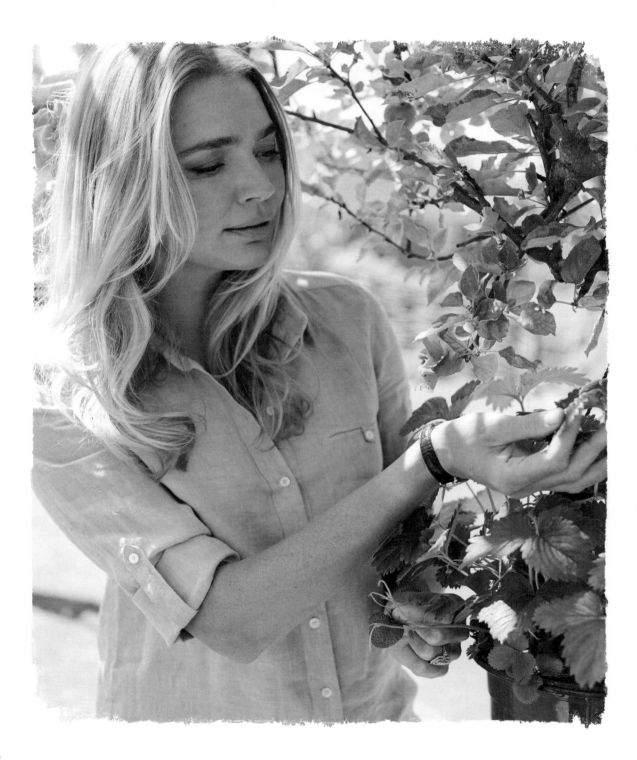

A few times I've failed and had a rich dessert or not done the exercise, but that's realistic. Don't beat yourself up. It's about balance. It's not all or nothing.

- Jodie

DAY 5

Breakfast

Choose from the selection on pages 24–25

Lunch

SALADE À LA GRECQUE

SERVES 1

For the salad

100g (3½oz) cherry tomatoes, halved

100g (3½oz) cucumber, chopped

30g (1oz) feta cheese, crumbled

3 slices cooked free-range turkey breast, chopped

For the dressing

1 tsp extra virgin olive oil

juice of ½ lemon

½ shallot, very finely chopped

½ tsp Dijon mustard, or to taste

salt and pepper

1 In a serving bowl, mix together the tomatoes, cucumber, feta cheese, and turkey.

2 In a separate small bowl or cup, whisk together all the dressing ingredients, seasoning well, until thoroughly mixed.

3 Drizzle the salad with the dressing, toss gently to coat, and serve.

Dessert

5 level tbsp soya yogurt

Snack

Choose a snack from the list on page 25
(optional, only if you're hungry)

Dinner

SALMON WITH CREAMED SPINACH

SERVES 1

150g (5½oz) wild salmon fillet

1 lemon slice

spinach (as much as you want)

30g (1oz) half-fat crème fraîche

salt and pepper

2 slices wholemeal bread

1 Preheat the oven to 200°C (400°F/Gas 6). Line a baking sheet with greaseproof paper. Put the salmon fillet on it and set the slice of lemon on top. Cook in the oven for 10–12 minutes.

2 Meanwhile, steam the spinach for about 4 minutes, or until it has just begun to wilt. Then tip it into a dry saucepan and stir in the crème fraîche. Season with plenty of salt and pepper.

3 Serve the salmon with the spinach and wholemeal bread.

Dessert

5 level tbsp full-fat plain yogurt with natural flavouring

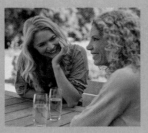

Jodie & Amélie

> **Amélie**
> What prompted you to want to make changes to your wellbeing in the first place?
>
> **Jodie**
> This year I've made it my goals to chase the mental clarity I've been seeking for years, realign my relationship with food, and go easier on myself.

DAY 6

Breakfast

Choose from the selection on
pages 24–25

pages 24–25

Lunch

LEMONY CHICKEN

SERVES 1

100g (3½oz) skinless,
boneless, free-range
chicken breast

extra virgin olive oil,
for brushing

pinch of ground cumin

2 garlic cloves,
finely sliced

1 lemon slice

salt and pepper

broccoli florets (as much
as you want)

1 Preheat the oven to 200°C (400°F/Gas 6). Brush the
chicken breast with oil and place in an ovenproof dish.
Rub the chicken all over with the cumin, scatter over
the garlic, and place the lemon slice on top. Season
to taste with salt and pepper.

2 Bake for 30 minutes, splashing in 5 tablespoons
of water after 10 minutes.

3 Meanwhile, steam the broccoli for about 5 minutes.
Serve with the chicken.

Dessert

Baked cinnamon apple (see page 33)

see page 33

Snack

Choose a snack from the list on page 25
(optional, only if you're hungry)

list on page 25

*"Always cook pasta
al dente, to minimize
sugar content (GI) and
keep your blood sugar
levels in check. "*

– Amélie

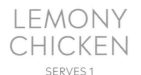

Penne primavera

40

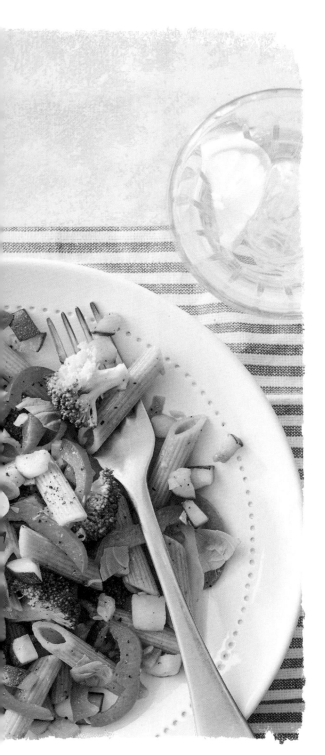

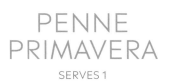

Dinner

PENNE PRIMAVERA

SERVES 1

100g (3½oz) wholegrain penne	small bowl of broccoli florets
1 tbsp extra virgin olive oil	1 courgette, finely chopped
1 garlic clove, crushed	salt and pepper
1 red pepper, finely sliced	small handful of basil leaves

1 Cook the penne according to the packet instructions, then drain and set aside.

2 Meanwhile, for the primavera sauce, heat the oil in a saucepan over a medium heat. Add the garlic, red pepper, broccoli, and courgette, season well, and sauté for about 5 minutes, or until tender.

3 Add the cooked pasta to a serving bowl, stir in the sauce, and serve sprinkled with basil leaves.

Dessert

Small bowl of cherries

DAY 7

On the last day of the week, build your own
food day, having your favourite meals
of the week from the list on pages 20–21.

Breakfast

Choose from the
selection on pages 24–25

Snack

Choose from the
selection on page 25

Lunch

Choose your favourite from
the week (see pages 26–41)

Dinner

Choose your favourite from the
week (see pages 26–41) or try one of
Jodie's own recipes on the following pages

Dessert

Choose your favourite from
the week (see pages 26–41)

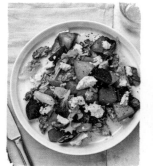 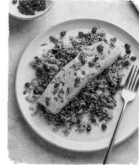

Dessert

Choose your favourite from
the week (see pages 26–41)

< WEEK 2

*Go back to page 26
and repeat*

*Continue on to
Phase Two (see page 82)*

WEEK 3 >

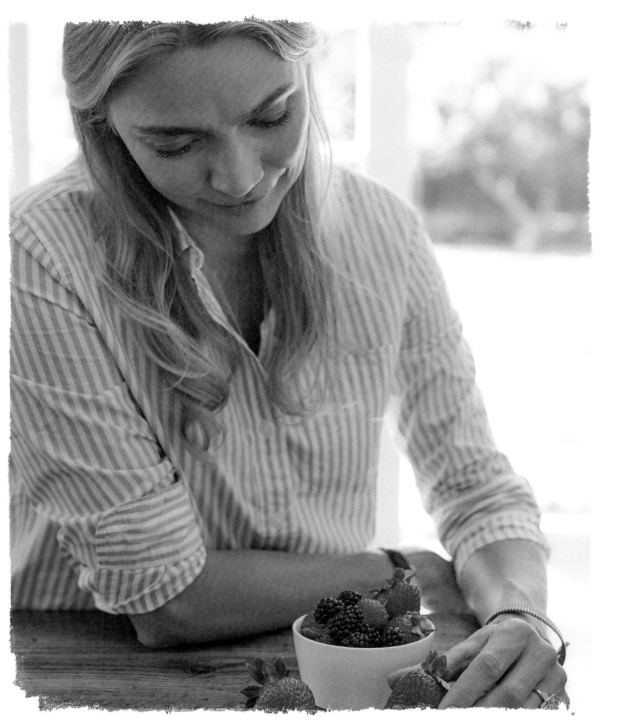

Jodie's recipe

ROAST BEETROOT SALAD WITH GOAT'S CURD

A feast for the senses, the rainbow of colours in this recipe is a sure sign that it will do you good. Use a combination of golden, candy stripe, and ruby beetroot to liven things up even further.

PREP 15 MINS
COOK 60 MINS
SERVES 2

6 small beetroot, about 250g (9oz) in total, including golden, candy stripe, and ruby, stalks trimmed

4 tbsp rapeseed oil, plus extra for drizzling

50g (1¾oz) walnut halves

2 tbsp runny honey

2 tbsp white wine vinegar

salt

60g (2oz) mixed salad leaves

85g (3oz) goats' curd, crumbled into bite-size chunks

1 Preheat the oven to 180°C (350°F/Gas 4). Arrange the beetroot in a small roasting tin. Drizzle each with a little rapeseed oil. Bake for 45 minutes, or until you can put a knife into them with no resistance. Remove from the oven, and when cool enough to handle, peel them. The skin should come off easily. Set the peeled beetroot aside.

2 Place the walnuts in a single layer on another baking tray, add to the oven, and roast for 5 minutes, shaking the tray occasionally so they cook evenly, until they are darker in colour and fragrant. Remove from the oven and set aside.

3 Add the honey and white wine vinegar to a bowl and whisk together to blend. Whisking continuously, add the remaining rapeseed oil in a thin stream until emulsified. Season with a little salt, if liked, and set aside.

4 Slice the warm beetroots into wedges. Place the salad leaves and walnuts in a large salad bowl.

5 Add the warm beetroot to the salad bowl, drizzle with the dressing, and toss together to coat. Divide the salad among serving plates, scatter over the goats' curd, and serve.

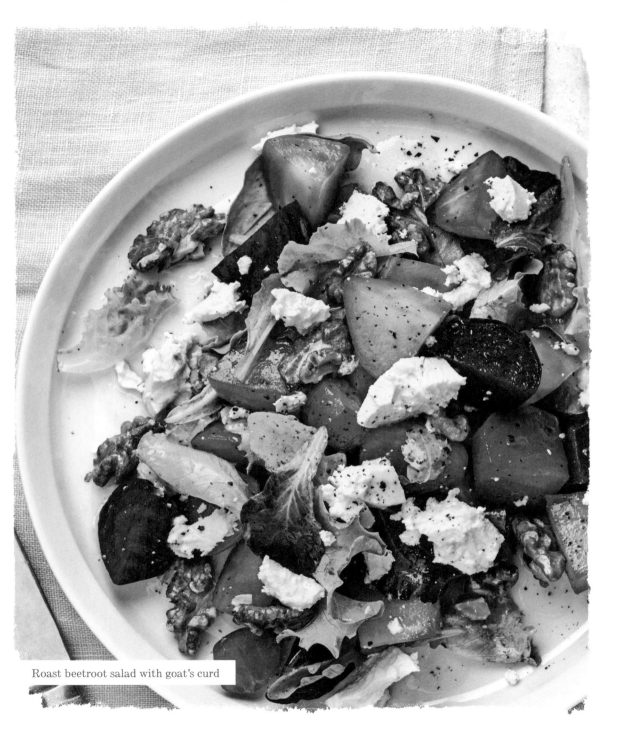

Roast beetroot salad with goat's curd

Jodie's recipe
POACHED SALMON ON QUINOA SALAD

This filling meal, rich in protein, is one to enjoy on a day when your resolve is waning. Stuffed full of nutrients and so colourful, this dish is absolutely bursting with flavour.

PREP 10 MINS
COOK 30 MINS
SERVES 2

600ml (1 pint) vegetable stock

600ml (1 pint) water

2 pieces of wild salmon fillet, about 175g (6oz) each, skin on

125g (4½oz) quinoa, rinsed under cold running water

1 tbsp rapeseed oil

4 spring onions, green and white parts, finely sliced

small bunch of coriander, leaves only, roughly chopped, plus extra to garnish

115g (4oz) baby leaf spinach rinsed and drained

seeds of ½ pomegranate, to garnish

1 Place 250ml (8fl oz) of the stock and the measured water into a shallow saucepan over a medium heat. Bring to the boil then reduce the heat to low. When barely simmering, submerge the salmon fillets in the liquid, skin-side up. Do not allow the liquid to boil. Poach for 5–6 minutes until cooked through. Remove the salmon with a slotted spoon and keep warm.

2 Add the quinoa to a saucepan over a medium heat and pour in the remaining stock. Cover and bring to the boil then reduce the heat. Leave to simmer for 20 minutes, or until tender and the stock has been absorbed. Remove from the heat but keep covered and warm.

3 Place the oil in a frying pan over a medium heat. Add the sliced spring onions and fry for 2 minutes. Add the spinach leaves to the pan and cook for 2 minutes, stirring until the leaves are wilted. Remove from the heat and stir them into the cooked quinoa with the chopped coriander.

4 Divide the quinoa mixture between two plates and place a poached salmon fillet on top of each. Sprinkle over the extra chopped coriander and pomegranate seeds, and serve.

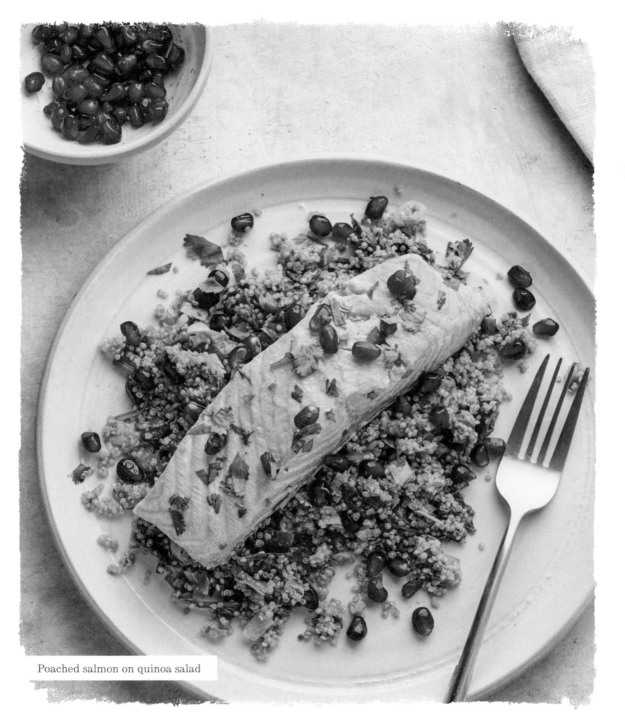

Poached salmon on quinoa salad

IGNITE
exercise plan

This is the 30-minute bodyweight-based exercise programme that you will follow over the next 2 weeks. It will kick-start the metabolic conditioning, burning fat while building muscle. You will need a timer. You can use an exercise mat to make the floor-based exercises more comfortable.

Work out with this routine 2 days in a row, then take a rest day to give your muscles a chance to recover and strengthen. Repeat working out two days in a row then taking one rest day for the full two weeks.

Speed is the essence of this workout. Proceed quickly from one exercise to the next, with a 15-second rest in between exercises, to give you the high level of intensity you need to see great results. The Warm up and Cool down do not have rests between exercises.

Make sure your posture is correct at all times, to avoid injuries and maximize results. Think about the movements you are performing and concentrate on the muscles that you are working and engaging.

Stay hydrated. Remember to drink water during your short rest breaks.

Stay in the moment and focus on each movement to make your body work harder and get results quicker.

WARM UP

INCHWORM (p50)

Repeat for 60 secs

SUMO SQUAT (p52)

Repeat for 60 secs

HIP AND BACK OPENER (p53)

Repeat for 60 secs

Weeks 1–2

COMPLETE WARM UP · COMPLETE SETS I & II · REST FOR 2 MINS
REPEAT SETS I & II ONCE MORE · COMPLETE COOL DOWN

SET I	SET II	COOL DOWN
SQUAT (p54) Repeat for 45 secs Rest for 15 secs	**ALTERNATED FORWARD LUNGES** (p66) Repeat for 45 secs Rest for 15 secs	**RUNNER'S LUNGE** (p78) Hold for 60 secs
MOUNTAIN CLIMBERS (p56) Repeat for 45 secs Rest for 15 secs	**PLANK JACKS** (p68) Repeat for 45 secs Rest for 15 secs	**BUTTERFLY** (p80) Hold for 60 secs
TRICEPS DIPS (p58) Repeat for 45 secs Rest for 15 secs	**MODIFIED PUSH-UPS** (p70) Repeat for 45 secs Rest for 15 secs	**LEGS UP WALL** (p81) Hold for 60 secs
JUMPING JACKS (p60) Repeat for 45 secs Rest for 15 secs	**HIGH KNEES** (p72) Repeat for 45 secs Rest for 15 secs	
WALKING LUNGES (p62) Repeat for 45 secs Rest for 15 secs	**CURTSY LUNGES** (p74) Repeat for 45 secs Rest for 15 secs	
HIGH PLANK (p64) Hold for 45 secs Rest for 15 sec	**ELBOW SIDE PLANK** (p76) Hold for 30 secs on each side Rest for 2 mins	
MOVE ON TO SET II	**REPEAT SETS I & II ONCE MORE**	

WARM UP

A mini exercise routine in itself, the Warm up should take 3 minutes. Don't skip it. Along with the Cool down (pp78–81), it is vital for your programme. Without it, you could succumb to injury, putting a halt to all your efforts.

Inchworm

Inchworm warms up all the muscle groups helping with mobility, strength, and flexibility. Good form is essential here in order to receive all the benefits, so perform this slowly.

WORK

Perform the exercise for 60 seconds, repeating as many times as you can.

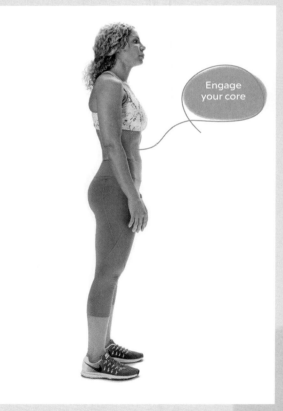

Engage your core

1 Stand with your feet hip-width apart and your navel pulled towards your spine.

2 Bend at the hips and place your hands on the floor. Walk your hands forwards, away from your feet.

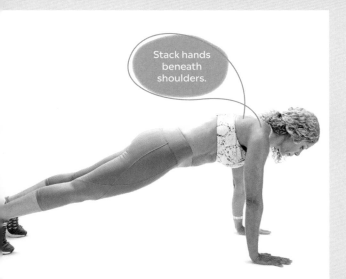

3 Continue until you come into a High plank (see p64), and pause briefly. If you feel the need to bend your knees, simply step your feet further apart. Try not to bend your legs.

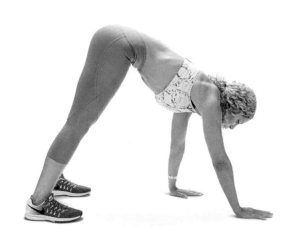

4 Walk your hands back towards your feet to return to the upright starting position. Repeat for 60 seconds.

PHASE ONE *weeks 1-2*

Sumo squat

Sumo squats are a low-impact exercise that help warm up the entire leg and bottom as well as the hip flexors, which tend to be tight.

WORK

Perform the exercise for 60 seconds, repeating as many times as you can. Focus on the stretch.

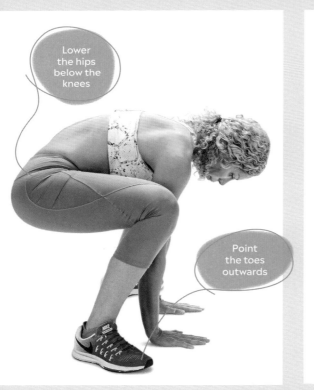

Lower the hips below the knees

Point the toes outwards

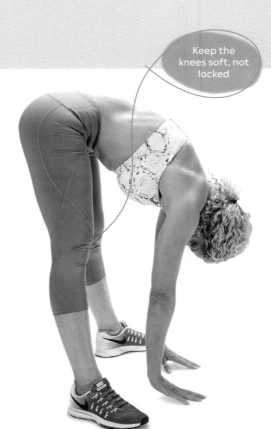

Keep the knees soft, not locked

1 Stand with your feet wider than hip-width apart, tailbone tucked in. Push your hips back and bend your knees to come into a low, wide squat. Place both hands flat on the floor.

2 Straighten both legs to come into a forward fold. Pause when you feel a stretch in the back of your thighs. Continue to squat and straighten your legs for 60 seconds.

Hip and back opener

This Warm up exercise helps open up the hip flexors, groin, and lower back and should be performed slowly. Keep your focus on the stretch you achieve from the depth of the lunge and the twist.

WORK

Perform the exercise for 60 seconds; alternating sides every 10 seconds.

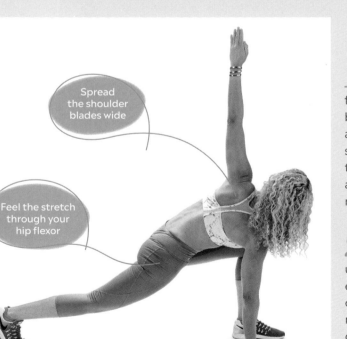

Spread the shoulder blades wide

Feel the stretch through your hip flexor

1 Start standing with your feet together. Take a big step forwards with your left foot and bend your left knee to drop into a lunge. Keeping your right leg straight behind you with your toes on the ground, so you feel a stretch at the front of your right thigh.

2 Place your right hand flat on the floor and twist your upper body to the left as you extend your left arm towards the ceiling. Hold for 10 seconds, then return to standing. Repeat on the opposite side. Continue to repeat the stretch, alternating sides, for a total of 60 seconds.

53

Squat

Squats are the cornerstone of any fitness routine, improving balance and coordination. They are a "compound exercise", meaning they engage the entire body. In my view it's just the best exercise: once you know how to squat you can do pretty much any other exercise.

WORK

Repeat the exercise for 45 seconds, then rest for 15 seconds.

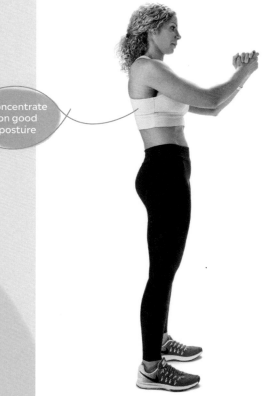

Concentrate on good posture

1 Stand with your feet hip-width apart. Clasp your hands together in front of your chest or – for a more challenging movement – put your hands behind your head.

*"The lower you go, the more
your glutes and lower abs work."*

- Amélie

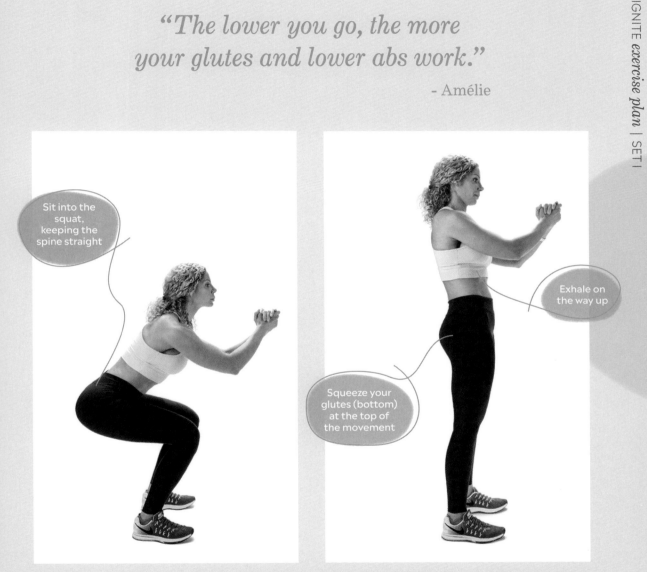

Sit into the squat, keeping the spine straight

Exhale on the way up

Squeeze your glutes (bottom) at the top of the movement

2 Keeping your weight in your heels, bend your knees, lowering your hips deeply so your thighs are parallel to the floor and your knees are no farther forwards than your toes. Inhale as you go down.

3 Press through your heels to rise back up, straightening your legs completely. Continue to repeat for 45 seconds.

55

PHASE ONE *weeks 1–2*

Mountain climbers

Here's an exercise that's good for both cardiovascular fitness and the core muscles. Mountain climbers recruit all of the upper-body muscles, working the abs, triceps, and shoulders. Depending on your speed they are like sprinting, but being performed in a plank position makes them low impact.

WORK

Perform the exercise for 45 seconds, then rest for 15 seconds.

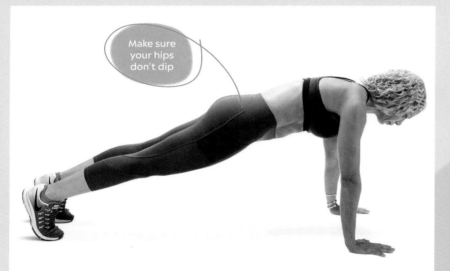

Make sure your hips don't dip

1 Start in a High plank (see p64) with your hands under your shoulders and your feet hip-width apart.

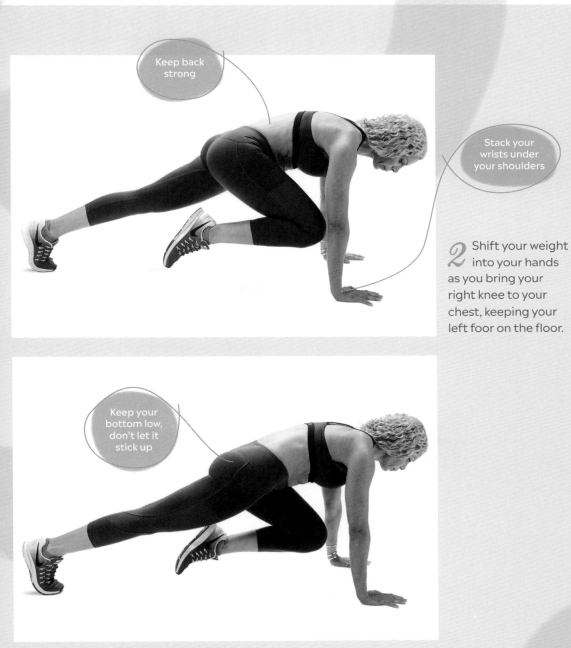

Keep back strong

Stack your wrists under your shoulders

2 Shift your weight into your hands as you bring your right knee to your chest, keeping your left foor on the floor.

Keep your bottom low, don't let it stick up

3 Switch legs quickly, bringing the left knee forwards while moving the right foot back into position, so that one foot replaces the other. Continue to repeat for 45 seconds.

57

Triceps dips

For this classic exercise it's very important to maintain good form. Make sure your elbows don't point outwards and don't let your shoulders rise up. Refrain from using your neck, and don't allow your head to move, otherwise, it takes away from the exercise and gives you a sore neck!

WORK

Perform the exercise for 45 seconds, then rest for 15 seconds.

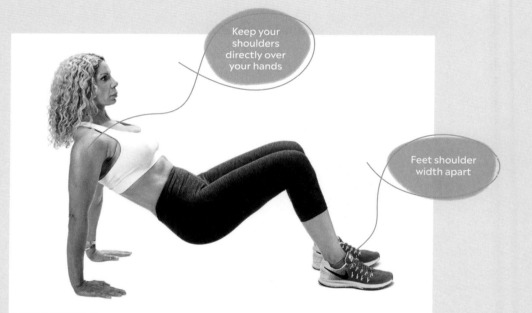

Keep your shoulders directly over your hands

Feet shoulder width apart

1 Sit on the floor with your hands behind you, shoulder-width apart and fingers pointing towards your feet. Position your feet away from your bottom. Straighten your arms and lift your pelvis.

Concentrate on using your triceps as opposed to your shoulders

2 Keeping your pelvis high, inhale, then bend your elbows so they stick straight out behind you. Don't let them point outwards to the sides.

Keep shoulders down - avoid hunching

3 Exhale while you straighten your arms, working the triceps. Continue to repeat Steps 2 and 3 for 45 seconds.

Jumping jacks

It's important to master this simple movement before you add speed to it. Keep the muscles in your core, arms, and legs engaged, and concentrate on your posture throughout.

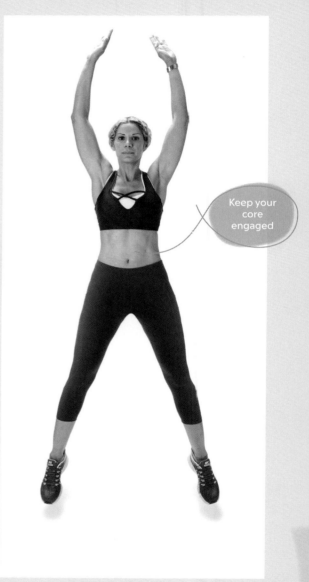

Keep your core engaged

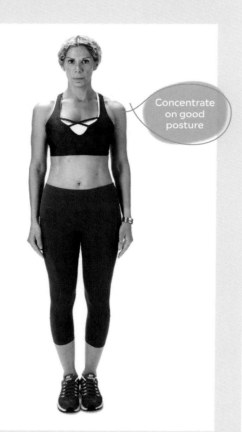

Concentrate on good posture

1 Stand tall with your feet together and your arms by your sides. Keep your knees soft and make sure your posture is good, with your navel drawn towards your spine.

2 Jump off the balls of your feet as you spread out your arms and legs to a wide star position. While your jump should be energetic, it should also be controlled.

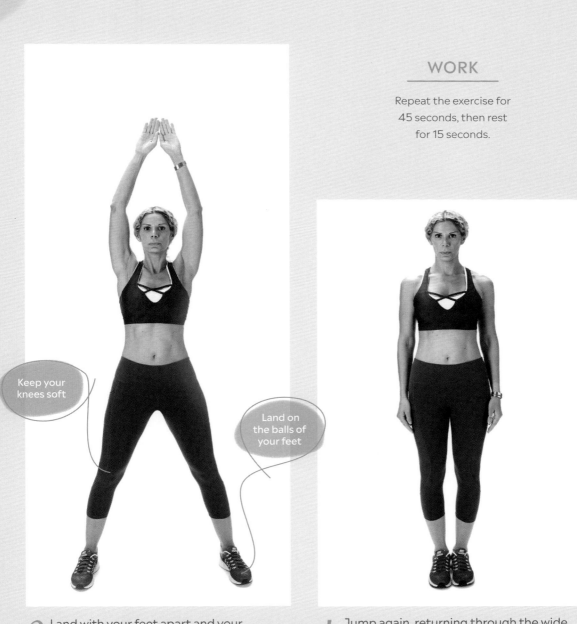

WORK

Repeat the exercise for
45 seconds, then rest
for 15 seconds.

Keep your
knees soft

Land on
the balls of
your feet

3 Land with your feet apart and your
hands touching over your head.

4 Jump again, returning through the wide
star position before landing with your feet
together and your arms by your sides, as in Step 1.
Repeat the exercise for 45 seconds.

Walking lunges

Form is everything, so don't try to go fast
here. The key is the depth of the lunge, not its
length, and to bring the back knee as close to
the floor as possible. The back leg does all the
work, helping you stabilize and control your
hips, core, and lower abs, as well as powering
that spring back up.

WORK

Repeat the exercise for
45 seconds, then rest
for 15 seconds.

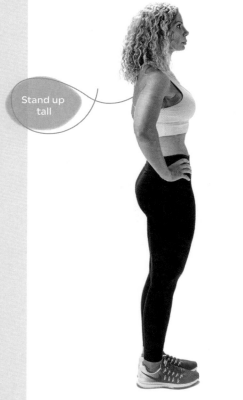

Stand up
tall

1 Stand tall with your feet together, your
shoulders back, and your hands on your hips.

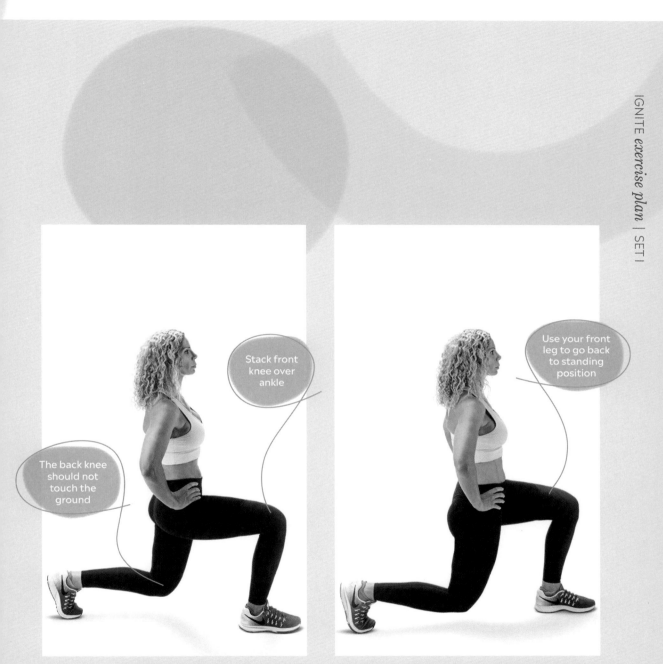

2 Take a controlled step forwards with your right foot, lowering your hips by bending both knees at right angles. The back knee should point towards the ground.

3 Press through your right foot and push off with your left foot to take a controlled step forwards with your left leg, down into a left lunge. Repeat Steps 2 and 3 for 45 seconds.

High plank

The holy grail of exercises, this is often performed poorly. Beginners should place their feet and hands wide apart for balance. If possible, practise in front of a mirror, or ask a friend to check your body is in a straight line from your tailbone to the top of your head.

WORK

Hold the plank for 45 seconds, then rest for 15 seconds.

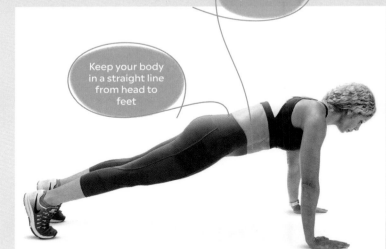

Pull your navel towards your spine

Stack your wrists under your shoulders

Keep your body in a straight line from head to feet

1 Crouch down with your palms on the floor, hands directly below your shoulders.

2 Walk your feet back until you are balancing on your hands and toes with your body in a straight line, hands under your shoulders and feet hip-width apart. Hold this position for 45 seconds.

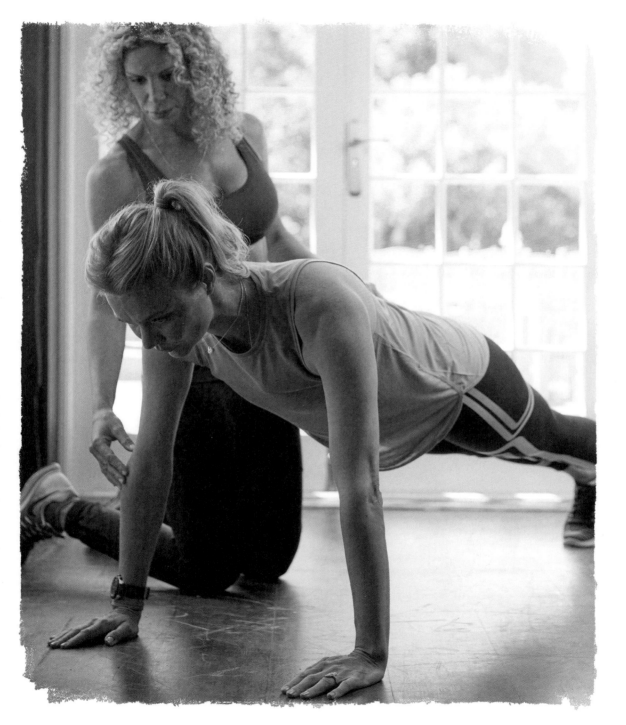

Alternated forward lunges

Take your time to focus and concentrate during this exercise, and think depth as opposed to length. Make sure you don't stay in the starting position for too long between lunges – you want to get your heart rate up.

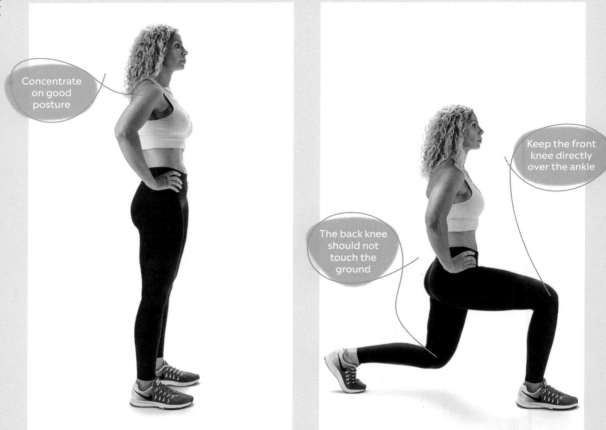

Concentrate on good posture

Keep the front knee directly over the ankle

The back knee should not touch the ground

1 Stand tall with your feet hip-width apart. Rest your hands on your hips, bending your elbows.

2 Take a controlled step forwards with your right foot, lowering your hips by bending both knees at right angles. The back knee should point towards the ground.

WORK

Repeat the exercise for
45 seconds, then rest
for 15 seconds.

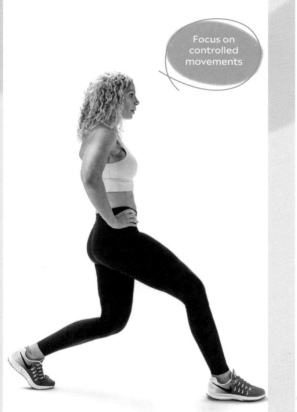

Focus on
controlled
movements

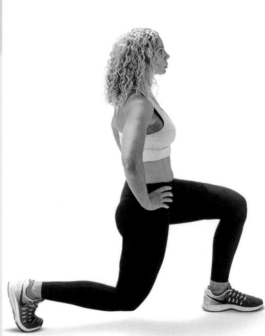

3 Keep your weight in your right heel as you push off with the right foot and straighten the right leg, back to the starting position (Step 1).

4 Repeat, this time stepping forwards with your left foot. Push back up through your left leg to the starting position. Repeat, alternating sides, for 45 seconds.

Plank jacks

Maintaining an engaged core at all times will help you perform this exercise correctly. Keep your hands wide and don't let your upper body dip between your shoulders. A lot of people tend to bounce around, dipping their bottom and hips. To avoid bouncing, focus on controlling your movement.

WORK

Repeat the exercise for 45 seconds, then rest for 15 seconds.

Pull your navel to your spine

Stack your wrists under your shoulders

1 Begin in a High plank (see p64), with your body in a straight line, hands placed under your shoulders, and feet together. Don't let your hips drop or your lower back arch.

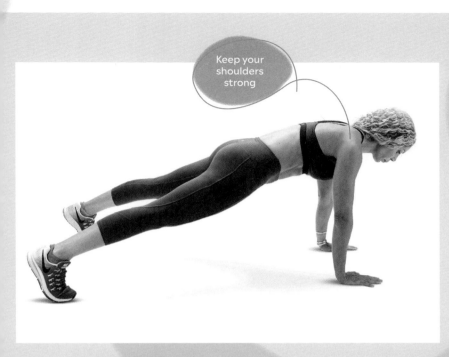

2 Jump your legs wide apart, keeping them straight and maintaining an engaged core.

3 Immediately jump your legs back together to return to the starting position. Repeat the exercise for 45 seconds.

PHASE ONE *weeks 1–2*

Modified push-ups

Technique is very important with this exercise. I often see people lowering themselves down while their hips and bottom stay up, but the body should be in a straight line from knees to head throughout the movement. Beginners should keep their hands wide.

WORK

Repeat the exercise for 45 seconds, then rest for 15 seconds.

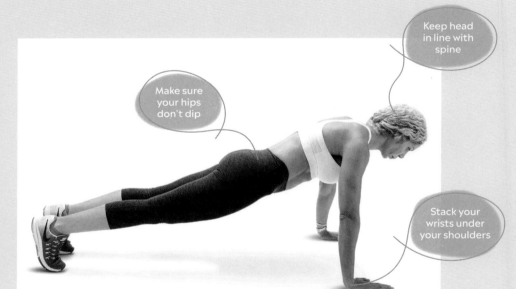

Keep head in line with spine

Make sure your hips don't dip

Stack your wrists under your shoulders

1 Start in a High plank (see p64), with your body in a straight line, hands under your shoulders, and feet together. Pull your navel towards your spine. Don't let your hips drop or your lower back arch.

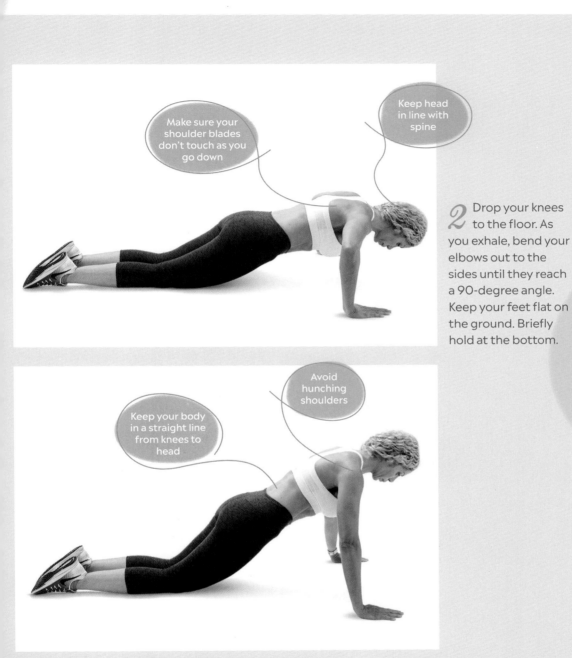

2 Drop your knees to the floor. As you exhale, bend your elbows out to the sides until they reach a 90-degree angle. Keep your feet flat on the ground. Briefly hold at the bottom.

3 Push through your hands to raise your torso up, but keep your knees on the floor. This completes one repetition. Repeat Steps 2 and 3 for 45 seconds.

71

High knees

This is not a sprint on the spot. Instead, you're aiming to get your knees to waist height and trying to stay on the balls of your feet. Don't hunch. It can help to put your hands, palms down, at waist height and aim to touch them with your thighs.

WORK

Perform the exercise for 45 seconds, then rest for 15 seconds

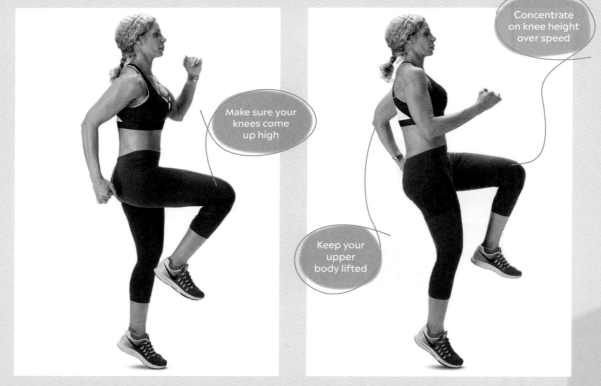

Make sure your knees come up high

Concentrate on knee height over speed

Keep your upper body lifted

1 Stand tall with your feet together. Begin to step on he spot by lifting your right knee high, to the level of your waist, engaging your core as the knee comes up. Pump your arms.

2 Lower your right leg back down, then raise your left knee, swinging ycur arms in the opposite direction. Repeat for 45 seconds.

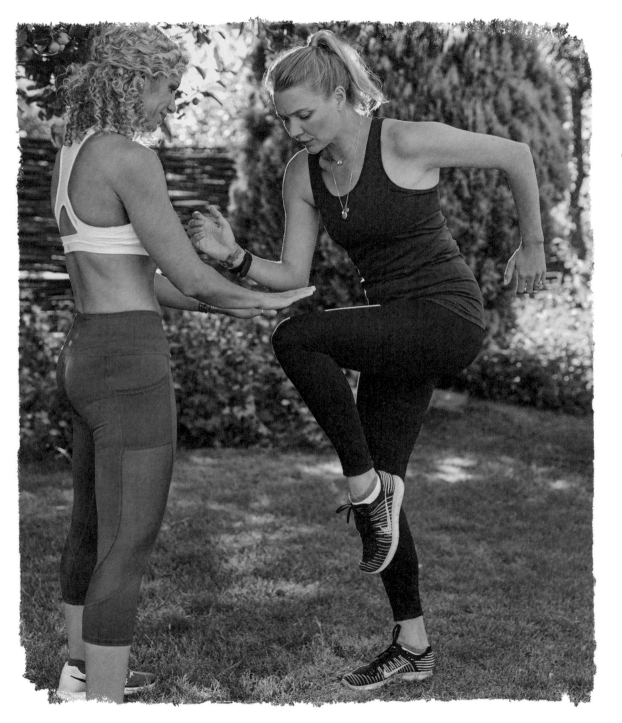

Curtsy lunges

This is a fantastic exercise to open up your hips, and to work your inner thighs, hamstrings, and the front of your thighs. It's the front leg that is doing all the work, even though the back leg is moving. The key is to place your back leg as far out to the side as possible, aiming for that knee to almost touch the floor.

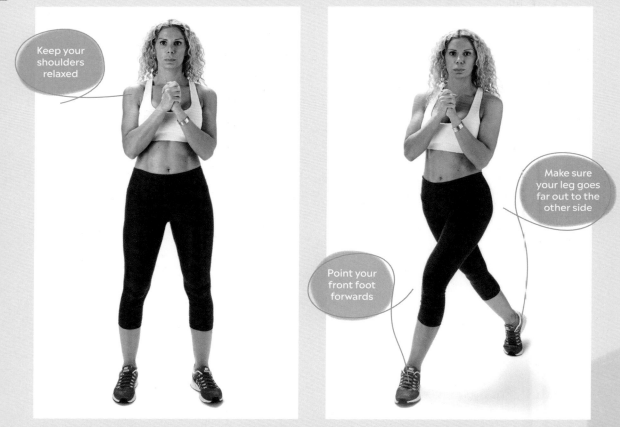

Keep your shoulders relaxed

Make sure your leg goes far out to the other side

Point your front foot forwards

1 Stand with your feet hip-width (or slightly wider) apart, chest up, and hands clasped together in front of you at chest height. Pull your navel towards your spine.

2 Lunge back diagonally with your right foot, crossing it behind your left knee.

WORK

Repeat the exercise for
45 seconds, then rest
for 15 seconds.

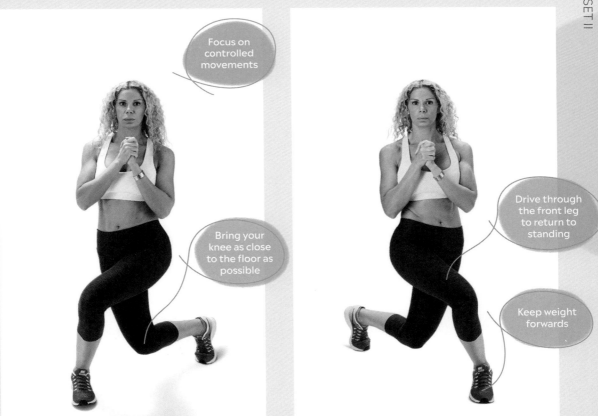

Focus on controlled movements

Bring your knee as close to the floor as possible

Drive through the front leg to return to standing

Keep weight forwards

3 Bend your knees (as if doing a curtsy) and lower your hips until your left thigh is almost parallel with the ground. Keep your navel pulled towards your spine and your chest up.

4 Push through the front leg to return to the starting position, then repeat on the other side. Repeat, alternating sides, for 45 seconds.

PHASE ONE *weeks 1–2*

Elbow side plank

Alignment is everything here. You can perform the exercise either with your feet stacked on top of each other, or you can have them staggered. Above all, it's important not to let your hips drop.

WORK

Hold for 30 seconds on each side.

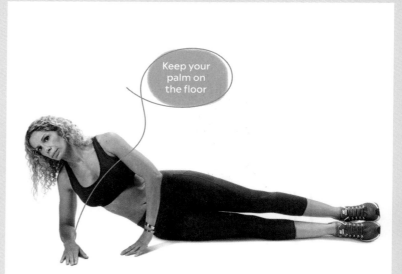

Keep your palm on the floor

1 Begin by lying on your right side, propped up with your right elbow directly under your right shoulder. Stack your heels, or stagger them if you need more stability.

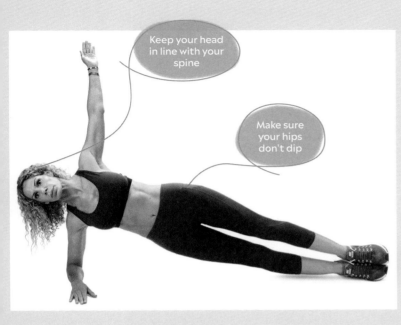

2 Engaging your core, press your right elbow into the ground, and use your core muscles to lift your torso and legs off the ground into a straight line. Reach your left arm up towards the ceiling, which will help you lift your waist. Hold for 30 seconds.

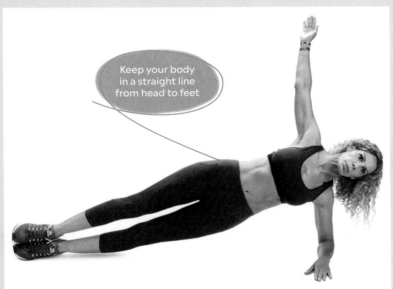

"If you feel pain in your lower back, bend the bottom leg and use it for support."
- Amélie

3 Lower your arm and your body back down, switch to the left side, and repeat on the left side, holding for 30 seconds.

COOL DOWN

This Cool down sequence will help to slowly bring down your heart rate and breathing. Do each of the movements for 60 seconds, with no rest in between, for a total time of 3 minutes.

WORK

Perform this stretch for 60 seconds.

Runner's lunge

The Runner's lunge is one of the best movements to stretch just about every muscle in your body. Don't be afraid to go far into the lunge, to really feel the stretch in your groin, but go gently. The depth you can achieve will improve with practise.

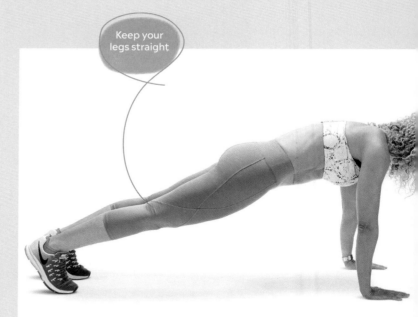

Keep your legs straight

1 Start in a High plank (see p64) with your hands directly under your shoulders and your body in one straight line.

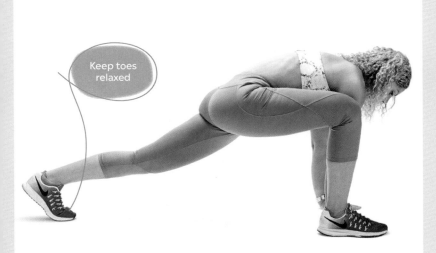

Keep toes relaxed

2 Step your right foot forwards so it sits to the outside of your hands. Your right knee should be at a right angle and your left leg extended behind you. Hold briefly, then repeat on your left side. Complete 10 lunges on each leg, swapping back and forth from side to side.

Butterfly

The Butterfly position stretches your groin, lower back, and – by using your elbows and arms to push your knees down – also your shoulders, opening your back. If you want an even deeper stretch, extend your arms out in front of you instead of holding onto your feet.

WORK

Perform this stretch for 60 seconds.

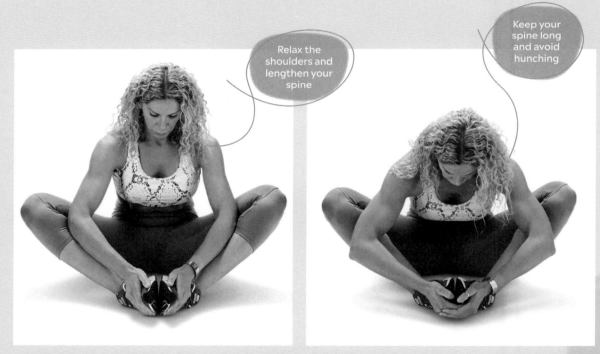

Relax the shoulders and lengthen your spine

Keep your spine long and avoid hunching

1 Sit on the floor, bring the soles of your feet together, and grasp them with your hands. Use your forearms to press your knees towards the floor. Look at your feet. Hold for 30 seconds.

2 Slowly begin to fold forwards, bringing your chest to your legs. Keep your hands on your feet, pressing your knees down with your arms. Hold for an additional 30 seconds.

Legs up wall

Legs up wall is a mind and body relaxer. Any movement where the legs are elevated will have a positive, relaxing impact on mood, as well as helping blood flow return to normal after a workout.

WORK

Perform this stretch for 60 seconds.

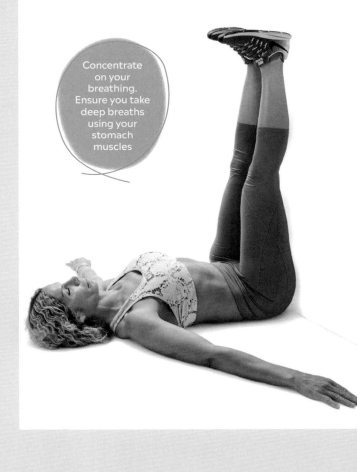

Concentrate on your breathing. Ensure you take deep breaths using your stomach muscles

1 Lie on your back and place your feet on a wall with your knees bent. Scoot your body over so your bottom is touching the wall. Straighten your legs, resting your heels on the wall. You can keep your arms extended on the floor at your side or behind your head (the latter position will stretch your shoulders).

2 Close your eyes and allow your entire body to relax. Be aware of gravity pulling you down as the wall supports you. Hold for at least 60 seconds, before rolling onto one side with your knees bent. Slowly sit up, then stand, before moving on with the rest of your day.

PHASE TWO

weeks 3–4

The next two weeks of the programme
will fight stubborn fat and help you
achieve stronger, more defined muscles.
It's broken down into a FIGHT EATING
PLAN and a 48-minute BODY TRAINING
EXERCISE PLAN. If you feel your
motivation waning, remember that you are
doing your body and mind a huge favour
by looking after them.

FIGHT
eating plan

This is the meal plan you will follow over the next two weeks. Once a week, on the day of your choice you will do a "Fire Fight Day". I suggest you pick your "Fire Fight Day" at the beginning of the week, and then stick to that plan. Like Phase One, on Day 7 you can build your own meal plan using the recipes from earlier in the week, or use one of Jodie's recipes.

Keep drinking the warm cinnamon water and lemon (see p12) first thing in the morning, even on the "Fire Fight Day".

Remember to drink 1.5–2 liters (2¾–3½ pints) of water each day, finish every day with a mug of herbal tea, and always take the time to sit down to eat.

You can pick your breakfast each day, as in Phase One, except for on your "Fire Fight Day".

You can choose one snack from the options on page 89 to have each afternooon. As with breakfasts, you can choose whichever snack appeals to you most.

The night before your "Fire Fight Day" I advise that you go on a screen detox from 9pm. Don't look at social media or your emails for the evening. This will allow you to sleep better and keep coritsol, a stress hormone, at bay. It also frees up some time to cook and meal prep for the week, if needed.

On Day 7 you can choose to make one of Jodie's recipes (see pp106–09) instead of repeating recipes from earlier in the week.

You will need a steamer, non-stick frying pan, and kitchen scales to hand.

BREAKFAST

LUNCH

DINNER

BREAKFAST

LUNCH

DINNER

BREAKFAST

LUNCH

DINNER

BREAKFAST

LUNCH

DINNER

Weeks 3–4

"FIRE FIGHT DAY"	DAY 2
Tea and 2 boiled eggs	Choose from the selection on pages 88–89
Superfood salad	Green salad with vinaigrette
Ratatouille Provençal	Notting Hill burger
DAY 3	**DAY 4**
Choose from the selection on pages 88–89	Choose from the selection on pages 88–89
Puy lentil and cucumber salad	Paprika chicken
Steak Provençal	Pesto turkey
DAY 5	**DAY 6**
Choose from the selection on pages 88–89	Choose from the selection on pages 88–89
Anise salad	Wholegrain penne, tuna, and chickpea salad
Marinated chicken with spiced rice	Coconut prawns

DAY 7	
Choose from the selection on pages 88–89	
Choose your favourite lunch recipe from the week, or try one of Jodie's recipes	
Choose your favourite dinner recipe from the week, or try one of Jodie's recipes	

A word on alcohol

You may be missing your regular evening drink, but it's important to remember the chemical effects alcohol has on your body and mind. Drinking leads to poor nutritional choices, which reduce your chance of success.

FIGHT
Weekly shopping list

Here's your list for Phase Two. Once again, every piece of meat, fish, or fruit, and all vegetables you eat must be organic. Remember also that, as with the Declutter Eating Plan, you will need to buy extra for Days 7 and 14, when you choose your favourite meals from the week to cook again, or choose one of Jodie's recipes, and for desserts, breakfasts, and snacks.

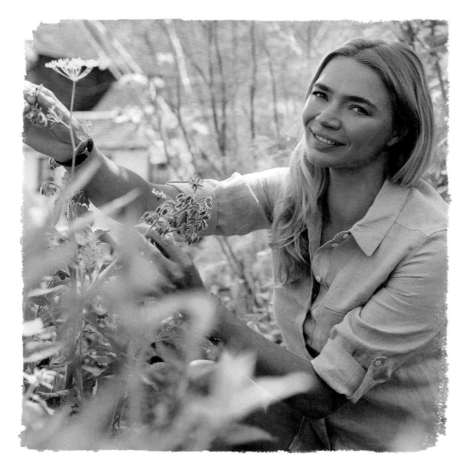

Fruits and vegetables

Apple 1
Granny Smith, Pink Lady, or Gala

Aubergine 1

Beetroot, cooked 1

Beetroot raw unlimited

Broccoli unlimited

Celery 3 sticks

Courgette 1

Cucumber unlimited, for salads, plus ½ extra

Fennel 1 bulb

Garlic 2 heads

Ginger, fresh root
small piece

Green beans, extra fine
unlimited

Herbs
Buy your herbs in bunches or packs.
You will need:
Basil
Coriander
Flat-leaf parsley
Mint

Lemons 7

Lettuce unlimited
Romaine, iceberg, rocket

Mushroom, Portobello
1 large

Onions 3

Pepper, green unlimited

Pepper, red 1

Shallot 1

Spinach 200g (7oz), plus
2 handfuls extra

Spring onions unlimited

Tomatoes, cherry
unlimited, for salads, plus
5 extra

Tomatoes, regular 3

Meat, fish, and eggs

Beef, minced (lean)
100g (3½oz)

Chicken breasts, raw,
free-range 2
140g (5oz) each

King prawns
150g (5½oz)

Salmon, smoked
100g (3½oz)

Steak, sirloin 1
200g (7oz)

Tuna in brine
160g can

Turkey breast, free-
range, raw
150g (5½oz)

Turkey, cooked
2 slices

Dairy and non-dairy alternatives

Cream, double
50ml (2fl oz)

Crème fraîche, half-fat
3 tbsp

Store cupboard

You'll still need some of
the supplies you bought
for Phase One, so keep
track of what you need
to top up.

Almond butter (crunchy)

Bay leaves, dried

Bouquet garni

Bread, rye, sourdough,
wholemeal

Caraway seeds

Chicken stock, organic

Chickpeas, canned

Cinnamon sticks

Coconut milk

Couscous, wholegrain

Cumin

Curry powder

Dark agave syrup

Extra virgin olive oil spray

Extra virgin organic
olive oil

Greaseproof paper

Herbes de Provence

Lentils, Puy

Mustard, Dijon

Oregano, dried

Pasta, wholegrain penne

Pesto

Rice, basmati brown

Rice, brown

Smoked paprika

Soy sauce, reduced salt

Tomatoes, canned
chopped

Tomato purée

Vinegar, balsamic

Vinegar, organic apple
cider

Beverage

Herbal tea
Any of your choice

Water, sparkling or still
You can choose either, as
long as you drink up to
1.5–2 litres (2¾–3½ pints)
every day

Breakfasts, snacks, and
herbal teas are all your
choice. Look through the
recipes (pp88–109),
decide what you'd like
to eat, and then shop
accordingly.

BREAKFASTS *and* SNACKS

Eat any of these breakfasts each morning during Weeks 3–4, apart from on your "Fire Fight Day" when you must have the "Fire Fight" breakfast (Option 1). If you are hungry after lunch, have one of the snacks opposite in the afternoon.

Breakfast options

Option 1
"FIRE FIGHT" BREAKFAST

HERBAL TEA
+
2 BOILED EGGS
(boiled to your liking)

Option 2

2 DARK RYE CRISPBREADS
+
½ SLICED AVOCADO
+
1 BOILED EGG
(boiled to your liking)

Option 3

RYE OR WHOLEMEAL SOURDOUGH BREAD
2 slices with a thin layer of almond butter
+
BLUEBERRIES
½ small bowl, or ½ mug

Snack options

Choose any one of these snacks to eat in the afternoon to bridge the gap between lunch and dinner. On your "Fire Fight Day" you must have snack Option 1.

Option 1

1 POT OF FULL-FAT PLAIN YOGURT WITH A CUP OF HERBAL TEA

Option 2

1 APPLE

Option 3

1 POT OF FULL-FAT YOGURT

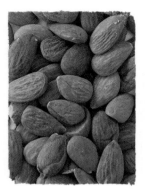
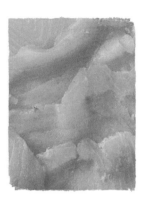
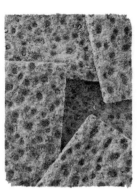
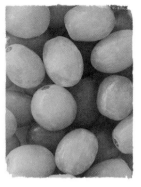

Option 4

OVERNIGHT OATS

The night before serving, half-fill a small bowl or a mug with rolled oats and just cover with water. Sweeten with 1 tsp agave syrup, if you like. Stir, cover, and refrigerate overnight.

+

10 ALMONDS
(add them to the oats, if you like)

Option 5

RYE OR WHOLEMEAL SOURDOUGH BREAD

2 slices with a thin layer of butter

+

2 slices smoked salmon

Option 6

COOKED FREE-RANGE CHICKEN

3 slices

+

10 ALMONDS

Option 7

EGG WHITE OMELETTE

Beat 2 egg whites in a bowl, adding a small handful of chopped soft herbs, if you wish. Place a frying pan over a medium heat and add ¼ tsp extra virgin olive oil. Pour in the egg whites and cook until set. Flip the omelette over to cook the other side.

+

2 DARK RYE CRISPBREADS
+
1 APPLE

Option 4

GREEN GRAPES
1 small bowl, or mug

Option 5

2 OATCAKES WITH ALMOND BUTTER

Option 6

2 BOILED EGGS
(boiled to your liking)

Option 7

2 SQUARES OF 70 PER CENT DARK CHOCOLATE WITH A CUP OF HERBAL TEA

DAY 1
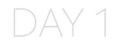

"FIRE FIGHT DAY"

Breakfast

"Fire Fight" breakfast (see p88)

Lunch

SUPERFOOD SALAD

SERVES 1

1 Romaine lettuce, chopped

1 medium beetroot, cooked and chopped

½ cucumber, chopped

4 cherry tomatoes, chopped

2 slices cooked free-range turkey, chopped

For the dressing

1 tsp extra virgin olive oil

juice of ½ lemon

salt and pepper

1 Put the chopped vegetables in a bowl with the turkey.

2 In a small bowl or cup, whisk the oil and lemon juice until thoroughly mixed, then season well with salt and pepper.

3 Drizzle the salad with the dressing and toss gently to coat.

Dessert

1 apple, or ½ small bowl berries

Snack

1 pot of plain yogurt and a cup of herbal tea (optional, only if you're hungry)

Dinner

RATATOUILLE PROVENÇAL

SERVES 1

1 tbsp extra virgin olive oil

1 onion, chopped

2 garlic cloves, crushed

1 aubergine, chopped

2 tomatoes, chopped

1 courgette, chopped

1 tbsp tomato purée

salt and pepper

2 slices wholemeal bread

For the bouquet garni

2 bay leaves

½ tsp thyme

1 Heat the oil in a large saucepan over a low heat. Add the onion and garlic and let them cook slowly for 8-10 minutes, until tender.

2 Add the rest of the vegetables along with the bouquet garni. Stir gently to distribute the ingredients evenly.

3 Dilute the tomato purée in 120ml (4fl oz) warm water and add to the saucepan. Season with salt and pepper, and stir well.

4 Cover and leave to cook for about 45 minutes, stirring occasionally. Remove the bay leaf. Serve warm with the wholemeal bread.

Dessert

½ mug of blueberries
peppermint or cinnamon tea, sweetened with
1 tsp agave syrup

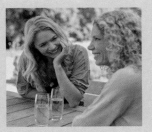

Jodie & Amélie

> ❝ ### Amélie
> Now in to Phase Two, how
> are you feeling?

Jodie
After two weeks it's becoming normal and easy
to do. I feel like I've started to form good habits
and that it's becoming a part of my everyday
way of life. With typical diets it can feel like
you're punishing yourself, but your approach
gives tools, not pressure. ❞

> ❝ ### Amélie
> It's drama-free. You're in charge, so you
> don't feel threatened. The more in control
> you are, the less impact the outside
> world has on you.

Jodie
I feel so much better for doing it,
and it's not asking too much from
my mind and body. ❞

DAY 2

Breakfast

Choose from the selection on
pages 88–89

Lunch

GREEN SALAD WITH VINAIGRETTE

SERVES 1

Romaine lettuce, or other
type of crisp lettuce of
your choice

1 green pepper, sliced

3–4 spring onions, sliced

For the dressing

1 tsp extra virgin olive oil

juice of ½ lemon,
or to taste

small handful of flat-leaf
parsley, leaves only,
chopped

salt and pepper

1 Add the salad ingredients to a serving bowl,
and toss together.

2 In a small cup or bowl, whisk the oil and lemon
juice until thoroughly mixed. Add the parsley and whisk
with a fork. Season well with salt and pepper.

3 Drizzle the salad with the dressing and toss
gently to coat.

Dessert

1 banana

Snack

Choose a snack from the list on page 89
(optional, only if you're hungry)

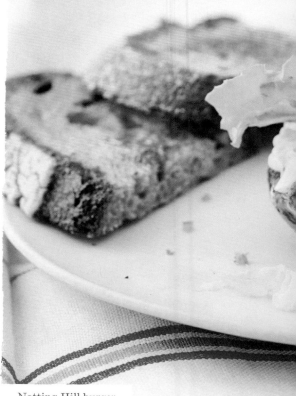

> *"Remember, it's all about balance. If you have a small lunch, you can balance it out with a more substantial dinner."*
>
> – Amélie

Notting Hill burger

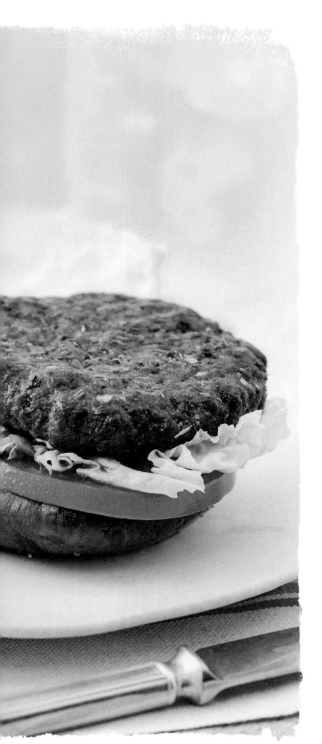

Dinner

NOTTING HILL BURGER

SERVES 1

100g (3½oz) lean
minced beef

1 garlic clove, crushed

1 tsp dried oregano

salt and pepper

1 large Portobello
mushroom

¼ tsp extra virgin
olive oil

To serve

1 tomato slice

2 lettuce leaves

1 slice rye bread
(optional)

1 Preheat the oven to 200°C (400°F/Gas 6). In a bowl, mix together the beef, garlic, and oregano, then season with salt and pepper. Shape the mixture into a patty, cover with cling film, and leave to chill in the fridge for about 15 minutes.

2 Place the mushroom on a piece of foil large enough to wrap around it. Drizzle with the olive oil, season with salt and pepper, and then fold the foil into a parcel. Place the parcel on a baking tray and cook for 20 minutes in the oven.

3 Meanwhile, remove the cling film from the burger and place it on another baking tray. Cook in the oven for 15–20 minutes, depending on how well done you prefer your meat.

4 Unwrap the mushroom and place it on your plate, topping it with the tomato slice, lettuce, and then the burger. Serve warm with the rye bread, if using.

Dessert

Small bowl of raspberries ,or
2 squares of 70 per cent dark chocolate

93

DAY 3

Breakfast

Choose from the selection on pages 88–89

Lunch

PUY LENTIL AND CUCUMBER SALAD

SERVES 1

100g (3½oz) Puy lentils

1 garlic clove, chopped

1 bay leaf

¼ cucumber, crushed

small handful of flat-leaf parsley, leaves chopped

For the dressing

1 tsp extra virgin olive oil

1 tbsp apple cider vinegar

juice of ½ lemon 1 tsp almond butter

salt and pepper

1 Rinse the lentils, put them in a medium-sized saucepan, and cover with cold water. Add the garlic and bay leaf and cook over a medium heat for 20 minutes, or until tender, then remove the bay leaf and drain.

2 Meanwhile, in a serving bowl, whisk together the olive oil, cider vinegar, lemon juice, and almond butter. Season with salt and pepper.

3 Add the lentils, cucumber, and parsley. Mix thoroughly and season with salt and pepper, to taste. Serve warm.

Dessert

1 apple

Snack

Choose a snack from the list on page 89

(optional, only if you're hungry)

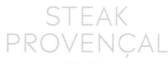

Dinner

STEAK PROVENÇAL

SERVES 1

100g (3½oz) wholegrain couscous

1 tbsp extra virgin olive oil

1 shallot, sliced

2 garlic cloves, crushed

1 tsp herbes de Provence

125g (4½oz) canned chopped tomatoes

1 bay leaf

salt and pepper

1 sirloin steak, about 200g (7oz)

extra-fine green beans, to serve

1 Prepare the couscous according to the packet instructions.

2 Meanwhile, heat half the oil in a saucepan over a medium heat and fry the shallot for 3 minutes, or until softened, stirring frequently. Add the garlic and herbs, and cook for 1 minute, stirring.

3 Stir in the chopped tomatoes and bay leaf and simmer over a low heat for 5–6 minutes, until reduced and thickened. Remove the bay leaf and season with salt and pepper to taste.

4 Meanwhile, heat the remaining oil in a frying pan. Season the steak and cook to your liking.

6 Steam the green beans for 3–5 minutes, or until tender but firm.

5 Serve the steak and couscous with the sauce spooned over the top and the green beans on the side.

Dessert

5 level tbsp full-fat plain yogurt

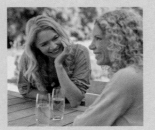

Jodie & Amélie

" Amélie

Let's talk about sleep for a minute. Are you strict about your sleep?

Jodie

I think anyone with a child gets used to sleep deprivation. I was surviving on probably five or six hours of sleep a night. "

" Amélie

Your brain doesn't function properly when it's sleep-deprived. It can have so many negative impacts.

Jodie

I'm now sleeping deeper and feeling more refreshed. I feel like the sleep I'm getting is of a better quality. "

Apparently, walking barefoot, in direct contact with the grass, can be good for you. Taking time to walk barefoot is one of the ways I've found to reduce my anxiety levels and reconnect.

– Jodie

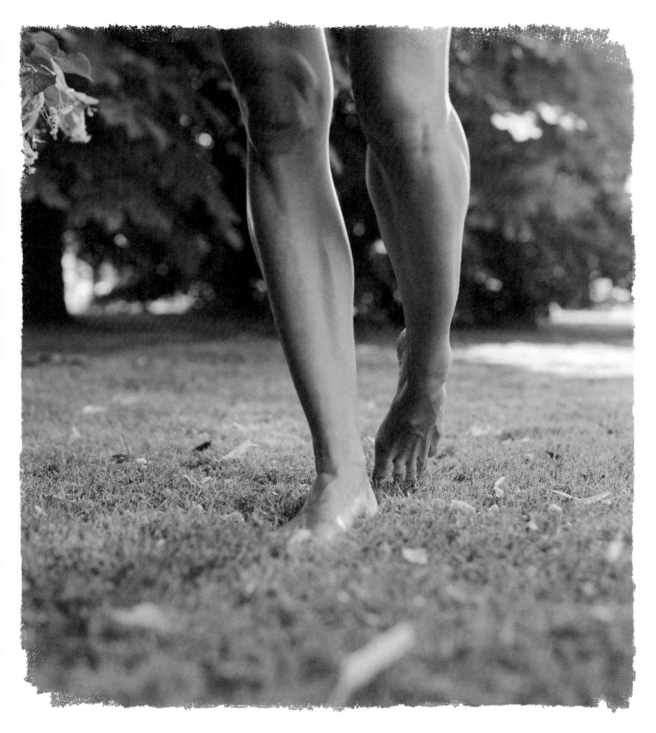

DAY 4

Breakfast

Choose from the selection on pages 88–89

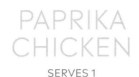

Lunch

PAPRIKA CHICKEN

SERVES 1

75g (2½oz) brown basmati rice

½ tbsp extra virgin olive oil

1 small onion, chopped

140g (5oz) skinless free-range chicken breast, chopped

small bowl of broccoli florets

1 garlic clove, crushed

½ tsp smoked paprika

½ tsp caraway seeds

1 tbsp half-fat crème fraîche

200g (7oz) spinach

1 Cook the rice according to the packet instructions.

2 Meanwhile, put the oil in a saucepan over a medium heat and gently cook the onion for 5 minutes, or until soft. Add the chicken breast and cook until golden.

3 Meanwhile, steam the broccoli for about 5 minutes.

3 Add the garlic, paprika, and caraway seeds to the chicken, and cook for a minute. Spoon in the crème fraîche, add the spinach, and cook for a further 2–3 minutes. Serve the rice and chicken with the steamed broccoli.

Dessert

Small bowl of blueberries

Snack

Choose a snack from the list on page 89 (optional, only if you're hungry)

Dinner

PESTO TURKEY

SERVES 1

1 free-range turkey breast, about 150g (5½oz)

salt and pepper

5 cherry tomatoes, halved

¼ cucumber, finely chopped

rocket (have as much as you like)

For the dressing

1 tsp pesto

½ tsp extra virgin olive oil

1 tsp balsamic vinegar

handful of basil leaves, roughly chopped

1 Preheat the oven to 200°C (400°F/Gas 6). Line a baking tray with greaseproof paper.

2 Cook the turkey on the prepared baking tray for 20–25 minutes, or until it is no longer pink on the inside when sliced. Season with salt and pepper, to taste, and allow to cool slightly.

3 In a serving bowl, whisk together the dressing ingredients and season with salt and pepper.

4 Add the turkey, cherry tomatoes, cucumber, and rocket, and toss gently to coat. Serve warm.

Dessert

1 apple

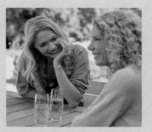

Jodie & Amélie

" ## Amélie
The mind-body relationship is a two-way street. Your mind is your ally, and what you put into your body will influence your mind.

Jodie
I always knew that "healthy body, healthy mind" was a thing, but now I feel it happening. **"**

" ## Amélie
Real, healthy food and exercise are not punishments.

Jodie
I'm finding that you reap the rewards from what you put in your body. I feel more positive and motivated and I have more energy. **"**

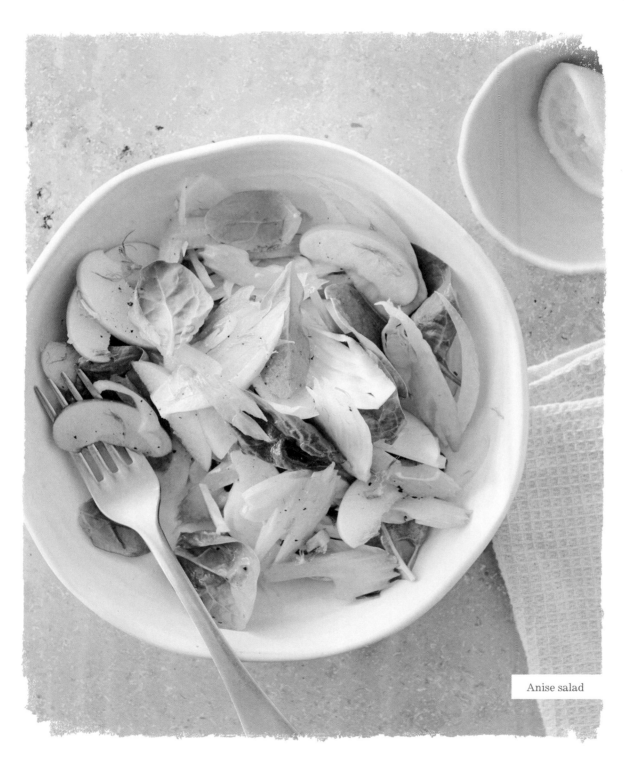

Anise salad

DAY 5

Breakfast

Choose from the selection on pages 88–89

Lunch

ANISE SALAD

SERVES 1

1 fennel bulb, finely sliced

2 celery sticks, finely sliced

handful of spinach

1 apple, finely sliced

For the dressing

juice of ½ lemon

1 tsp extra virgin olive oil

salt and pepper

1 Place all the vegetables and the apple into a bowl and set aside.

2 In a small bowl or a cup, whisk together the lemon juice and oil until thoroughly mixed. Season with salt and pepper, to taste.

3 Drizzle the salad with the dressing and toss gently to coat.

Dessert

5 level tbsp soya yogurt

Snack

Choose a snack from the list on page 89 (optional, only if you're hungry)

Dinner

MARINATED CHICKEN WITH SPICED RICE

SERVES 1

1 free-range chicken breast, about 140g (5oz)

½ tsp extra virgin olive oil

½ onion, chopped

1 garlic clove, crushed

100g (3½oz) brown rice

100ml (3½fl oz) chicken stock

2 bay leaves

1 cinnamon stick

salt and pepper

2 tbsp chopped coriander

2 tbsp chopped mint leaves

1 tbsp chopped basil leaves

For the marinade

50ml (1¾fl oz) double cream

finely grated zest and juice of ½ lemon

1 garlic clove, crushed

small piece of fresh root ginger, peeled and grated

¼ tsp curry powder

1 Whisk together the marinade ingredients in a bowl. Make a few cuts in the chicken breast and add to the marinade. Chill for a few hours, or overnight.

2 Preheat the oven to 200°C (400°F/Gas 6). Line a baking tray with greaseproof paper. Remove the chicken from the fridge and set aside until it is room temperature.

3 Scrape the chicken clean and place it on the prepared tray. Bake the chicken for 15 minutes.

4 In a saucepan, heat the olive oil over a low heat and add the onion and remaining garlic. Fry for 2 minutes, then add the rice and fry for 2 minutes more, stirring. Add the stock, bay leaves, and cinnamon stick, and season. Cover and cook for 30–40 minutes, or until the liquid has been absorbed. Remove from the heat, remove the bay leaves and cinnamon stick, and add the herbs. Serve warm with the chicken.

Dessert

Small bowl of raspberries with 1 crushed square of 70 per cent dark chocolate scattered over them

DAY 6

Breakfast

Choose from the selection on pages 88–89

Lunch

WHOLEGRAIN PENNE, TUNA, AND CHICKPEA SALAD

SERVES 1

100g (3½oz) wholegrain penne

½ red pepper, finely chopped

200g (7oz) canned chickpeas, drained and rinsed

160g can tuna in brine

1 celery stick, finely chopped

juice of 1 lemon

1 tsp extra virgin olive oil

salt and pepper

1 Cook the pasta according to the packet instructions. Drain and leave to cool.

2 When cooled, put the pasta in a serving bowl with the pepper, chickpeas, tuna, and celery, and set aside.

3 In a small bowl or cup, whisk together the lemon juice and oil until thoroughly mixed. Season to taste.

4 Drizzle the salad with the dressing and toss thoroughly to coat.

Dessert

Small bowl of green grapes

Snack

Choose a snack from the list on page 89
(optional, only if you're hungry)

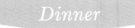

Dinner

COCONUT PRAWNS

SERVES 1

100g (3½oz) brown basmati rice

1 tsp extra virgin olive oil

1 small onion, finely chopped

green beans

150g (5½oz) king prawns

2 tbsp coconut milk*

¼ tsp curry powder

1 Cook the rice according to the packet instructions.

2 Meanwhile, heat the oil in a frying pan over a low heat and fry the onion for about 4 minutes, or until soft.

3 While the rice and onion are cooking, steam the green beans for 3–5 minutes, until firm but tender.

3 Add the prawns to the onion and cook until they are pink all over. Spoon in the coconut milk and curry powder. Serve over the rice with the green beans on the side.

Dessert

5 level tbsp full-fat plain yogurt

* Coconut milk does not freeze well, but you can store any leftover coconut milk for 4–6 weeks in the fridge. Simply transfer to a clean container and seal securely.

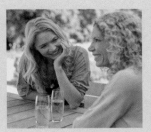

Jodie & Amélie

Amélie
Do you feel that doing regular exercise has changed your thinking on food?

Jodie
Because I've put effort in and am taking pride in what I'm doing, I don't want to throw it away with all the horrible naughty foods. I've been putting the time into my body, and it doesn't want these things.

Amélie
Your mindset starts to change.

Jodie
When I eat sugary food or drink wine I can feel it more strongly now – I get bloated and heavy. It feels like my body is telling me more about what it wants. I'm not interested in these things anymore.

Amélie
We talk about things like getting a sugar rush in children, but it's the same thing for adults.

Jodie
My whole household is doing it with me now, and not reluctantly either. Everyone is really happy moving in this direction with me. My dad still likes his glass of wine though!

DAY 7

As with the previous phase, use Days 7 and 14 to learn how to build your own optimum nutritional plan. If you want to boost weight loss, use this final day of the week as a second "Fire Fight Day".

Breakfast

Choose from the
selection on pages 88–89

Snack

Choose from the
selection on page 89

Lunch

Choose your favourite from
the week (see pp90–103)

Dinner

Choose your favourite from the
week (see pp90–103) or try one of Jodie's own
recipes on the following pages

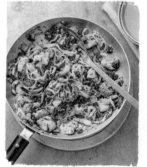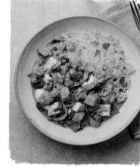

Dessert

Choose your favourite from
the week (see pp90–103)

Dessert

Choose your favourite from
the week (see pp90–103)

WEEK 3   *Go back to page 90
and repeat*

*Continue on to Phase
Three (see p140)*   WEEK 4

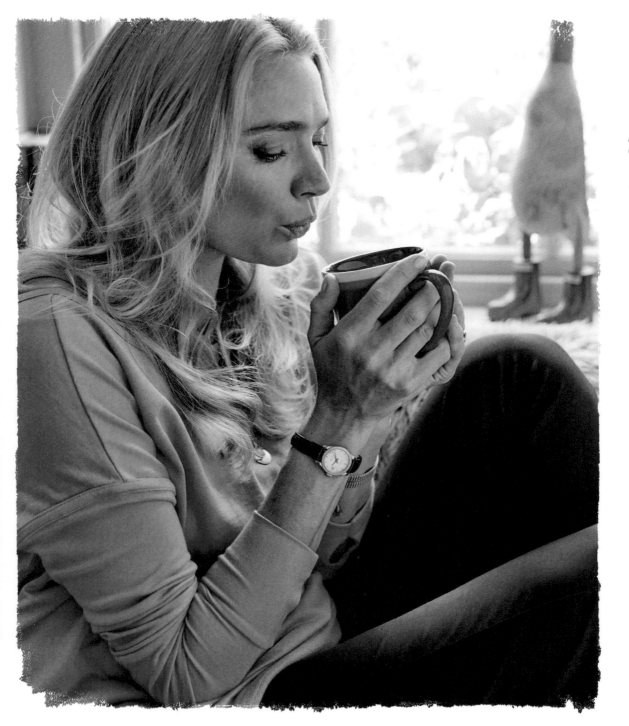

Jodie's recipe

CHICKEN STIR-FRY WITH GOJI BERRIES AND SEEDS

This stir-fry gives you a healthy range of ingredients – from tangy goji berries to earthy mushrooms – so you know you've got your daily nutritional needs covered. Best of all, it's quick and easy to prepare.

PREP 10 MINS, PLUS SOAKING
COOK 15 MINS
SERVES 2

100g (3½oz) folded dried rice noodles

45g (1½oz) fresh root ginger, peeled and roughly chopped

45g (1½oz) garlic, peeled and roughly chopped

1 tbsp rapeseed oil

2 shallots, sliced

2 skinless, boneless free-range chicken breasts, about 140g (5oz)each, diced

140g (5oz) mixed mushrooms, such as shiitake, chestnut, or exotic mushrooms, roughly chopped

2 pak choi, sliced

30g (1oz) chia seeds

30g (1oz) flax seeds

30g (1oz) goji berries

1 Place the noodles in a heatproof bowl. Add enough boiling water to cover the noodles. Set them aside to soak for 10 minutes.

2 Place the ginger and garlic in a blender and whizz to a paste. Set this aside while you heat the rapeseed oil in a large frying pan or wok over a medium heat.

3 Add the garlic and ginger paste to the oil and fry for 1 minute. Now add the shallots and stir-fry for 2 minutes, until soft.

4 Raise the heat to high, add the diced chicken, and stir-fry until the meat is coated with the paste, cooked through, and no longer pink. Add the mushrooms, pak choi, and the seeds and berries. Stir-fry them for 3 minutes, or until the mushroom and pak choi are cooked through.

5 Drain the noodles and add them to the pan or wok along with a little water, if liked. Toss all of the ingredients together and heap into bowls to serve.

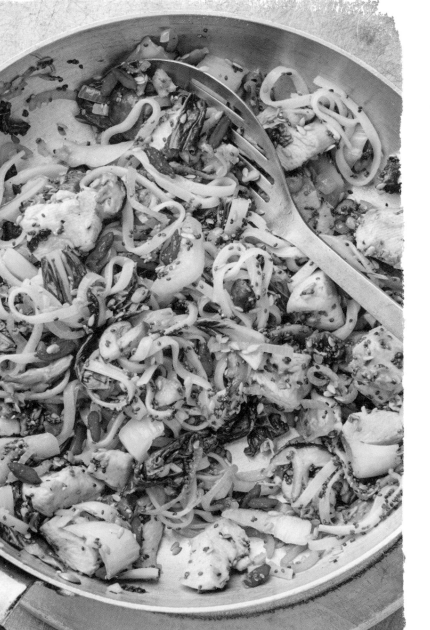

Chicken stir-fry with goji berries and seeds

Jodie's recipe
PANEER AND SWEET POTATO CURRY

The mouth-filling spices here hit every tastebud in a profoundly satisfying way. This recipe makes a lot of food, so halve the quantities if you're cooking for a smaller number. As a variation, you can use 300g (10oz) pollack or other white sustainable fish instead of the paneer.

PREP 15 MINS
COOK 15 MINS
SERVES 2

30g (1oz) fresh root ginger, peeled and roughly chopped

30g (1oz) garlic, peeled and roughly chopped

1 tbsp rapeseed oil

2 tsp ground turmeric

1 onion, sliced

2 sweet potatoes, peeled and diced (400g/14oz)

1 x 400ml can coconut milk

100g (3½oz) brown basmati rice

200g (7oz) paneer, cut into bite-sized cubes

85g (3oz) baby leaf spinach, rinsed and drained

salt and pepper

20g (¾oz) chopped coriander, to garnish

1 Place the ginger and garlic in a blender and whizz to a paste. Set this aside while you heat the rapeseed oil in a large frying pan or saucepan over a medium–low heat. Add the garlic and ginger paste and fry for 1–2 minutes.

2 Add the turmeric to the pan and cook for 30 seconds to release its spicy flavour. Now add the onion and stir-fry for 2–3 minutes, until soft.

3 Raise the heat to medium and add the diced sweet potatoes, stirring them to coat in the spice mixture. Pour in the coconut milk and 150ml (¼ pint) water. Leave this to simmer gently while you cook the rice according to the packet instructions.

4 Once you can slide a knife into a potato with no resistance, gently stir in the cubed paneer and the spinach. Leave to cook for 2–3 minutes, or until the paneer is cooked through and the spinach has wilted. Season to taste.

5 When the rice is cooked, drain it and divide it among two serving plates. Ladle the paneer curry either over the top or place it alongside the rice. Sprinkle over chopped coriander to garnish, and serve.

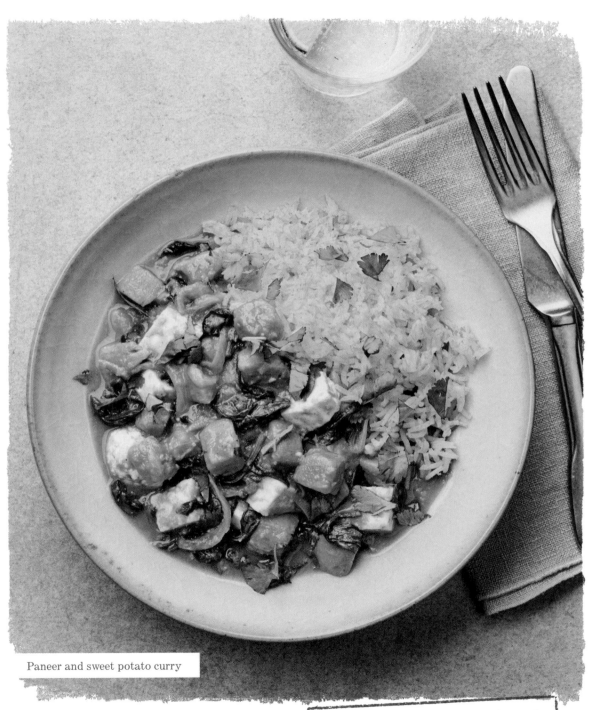

Paneer and sweet potato curry

BODY TRAINING
exercise plan

As well as burning fat, this 48-minute programme will help you achieve muscle definition and make you stronger physically and mentally. You will need a timer and two 2–3kg (4½–6½lb) dumbbells. You may also wish to have an exercise mat.

Work out with this routine every other day for the two-week phase.

Do three sets of each combo with a 60 second rest in between each set, then move onto the next combo. Do each exercise for 60 seconds.

Your Warm up is Combo I.

Make sure that your posture is correct at all times, to avoid injuries and maximize results. Think about the movements you are performing and concentrate on the muscles that you are working and engaging.

Remember to stay hydrated. Keep a water bottle close to your exercise mat and drink from it frequently during the short rest breaks. After working out, bear in mind that you will still need to top up with water regularly, to replace lost stocks and maximize the benefits for your muscles.

Stay in the moment and focus on each movement to make your body work harder and get results quicker.

COMBO I

REVERSE LUNGE AND SHOULDER PRESS (p112)

Repeat for 60 secs

RUSSIAN TWIST (p114)

Repeat for 60 secs

OVERHEAD TRICEPS EXTENSION (p116)

Repeat for 60 secs

BURPEES (p118)

Repeat for 60 secs

Rest for 60 secs

REPEAT COMBO I, INCLUDING REST, TWICE MORE

MOVE ON TO COMBO II

Weeks 3–4

COMPLETE COMBO I THREE TIMES · COMPLETE COMBO II THREE TIMES ·
COMPLETE COMBO III THREE TIMES · COMPLETE COOL DOWN

COMBO II	COMBO III	COOL DOWN
SUMO SQUAT WITH BICEPS CURLS (p120)	**SQUAT, CURL, AND PRESS** (p128)	**HAPPY BABY** (p136)
Repeat for 60 secs	Repeat for 60 secs	Hold for 60 secs
V-SITS (p122)	**SCISSORS** (p130)	**HEAD TO KNEE** (p137)
Repeat for 60 secs	Repeat for 60 secs	Hold for 60 secs
BENT-OVER ROW (p124)	**LYING CHEST FLY** (p132)	**TRICEPS STRETCH** (p138)
Repeat for 60 secs	Repeat for 60 secs	Hold for 60 secs
JUMP SQUATS (p126)	**PLANK JACKS** (p134)	
Repeat for 60 secs	Repeat for 60 secs	
Rest for 60 secs	Rest for 60 secs	
REPEAT COMBO II, INCLUDING REST, TWICE MORE	**REPEAT COMBO III, INCLUDING REST, TWICE MORE**	
MOVE ON TO COMBO III	**MOVE ON TO THE COOL DOWN**	

Reverse lunge and shoulder press

It's important to make sure your actions here are controlled. Keeping your core muscles engaged at all times will stabilize movements.

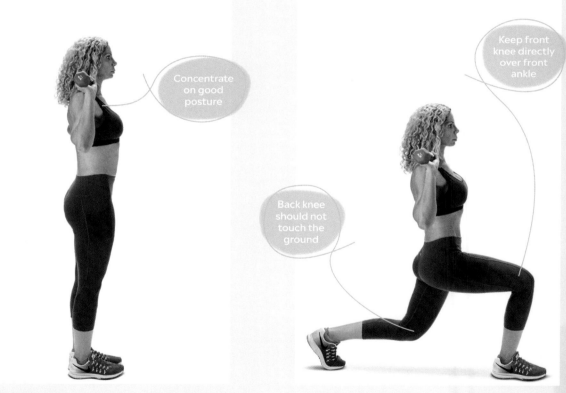

Concentrate on good posture

Keep front knee directly over front ankle

Back knee should not touch the ground

1 Stand tall with your feet together. Hold the dumbbells at shoulder height, with your palms facing slightly upwards.

2 Step your left foot back to come down into a lunge The back knee should point towards the ground. Focus on achieving depth, not length.

112

WORK

Repeat this exercise for
60 seconds (approximately
15 repetitions), alternating sides.

*"To remain balanced,
engage your core and fix your
gaze on a static point."*

- Amélie

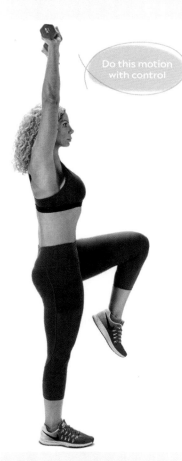

Do this motion
with control

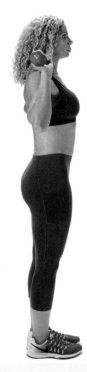

3 Pushing off with your left foot, bring your
knee up and forwards until it is at the same
height as your waist. At the same time, raise
your arms straight above your head.

4 Return to the starting position. To repeat,
step back into a lunge again, this time with
your right foot behind you. Perform this
exercise for 60 seconds, alternating sides.

Russian twist

For maximum effect when you're twisting side to side, keep your eyes on your hands. This way, both your gaze and your head follow your movements, increasing your upper-body stability.

WORK

Repeat this exercise for 60 seconds (approximately 15 repetitions), alternating sides.

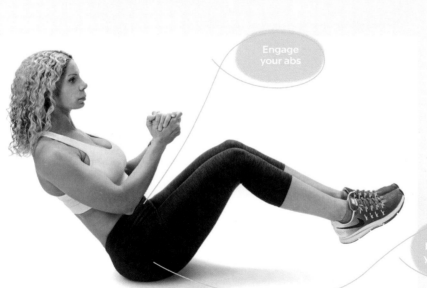

Engage your abs

Sit on your bottom, not on your lower back

1 Sit on the ground with your knees bent. Pull your abs towards your spine, then lean back a few centimetres while lifting your feet off the floor. Be sure to keep your back straight. Clasp your hands in front of you with your elbows bent.

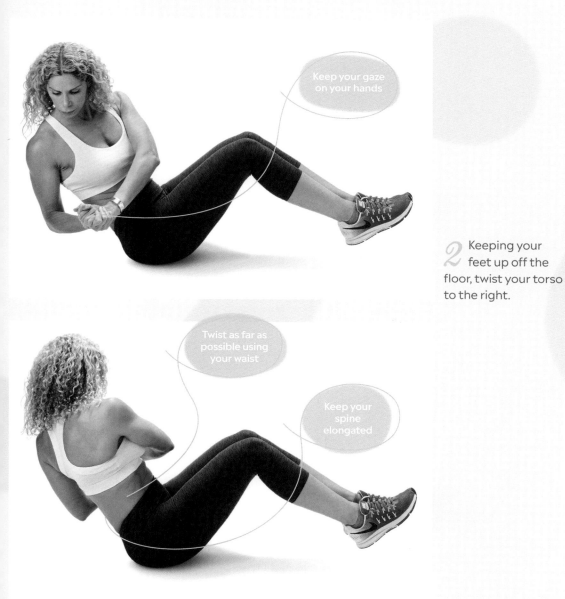

Keep your gaze
on your hands

Twist as far as
possible using
your waist

Keep your
spine
elongated

2 Keeping your
feet up off the
floor, twist your torso
to the right.

3 Then twist your torso to the left, before returning to
centre. This completes one repetition. Perform this
exercise for 60 seconds. To make it easier, you can lower
your heels to the ground if you need to.

Overhead tricep extensions

Do the movement slowly and smoothly so you can feel the burn in those triceps. There's no need to rush here.

WORK

Repeat this exercise for 60 seconds (approximately 15 repetitions).

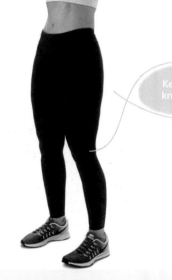

Keep your elbows very close to your ears

Keep your knees soft

1 Stand with your feet hip-width apart. Tuck your tailbone in. A slight bend in your knees will keep them soft. Hold one dumbbell with both hands above your head.

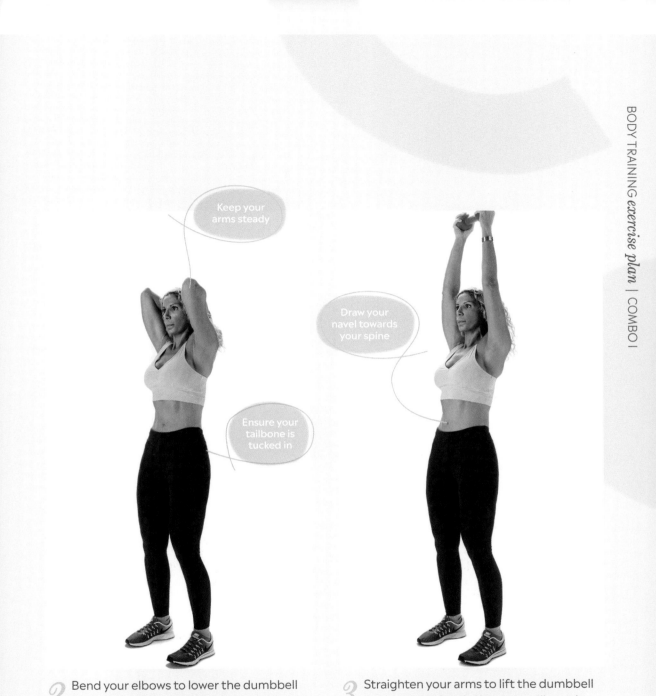

Keep your arms steady

Draw your navel towards your spine

Ensure your tailbone is tucked in

2 Bend your elbows to lower the dumbbell behind your head, keeping your elbows in line with your ears. Don't let your back arch as you move your arms.

3 Straighten your arms to lift the dumbbell back up into the air. Keep your elbows in line with your ears throughout. Repeat for 60 seconds.

Burpees

Super-technical, and my favourite exercise in the entire world. The key is to control your movements at all times by using your core – it is doing 70 per cent of the work here. Don't slam down on your hands or hips or you will just hurt yourself.

WORK

Repeat this exercise for 60 seconds (approximately 15 repetitions).

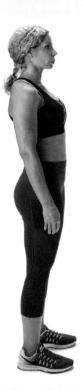

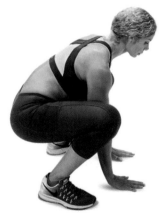

1 Stand tall with your toes angled slighty outwards and tailbone tucked in.

2 Step ypur feet slightly wider than wip-hidth apart. Push your hips back, and bend your knees to come into a low, wide squat. Place your hands on the floor.

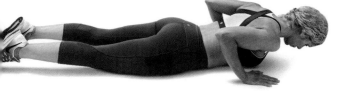

3 Jump your feet back into a High plank (see p64); your hands should be under your shoulders and your feet hip-width apart.

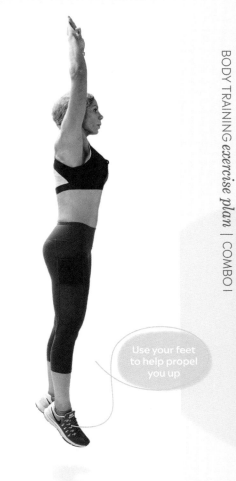

Use your feet to help propel you up

4 Bend your elbows to bring your chest as close to the floor as possible, then straighten them and lift your body back into a High plank.

5 Jump your feet towards your hands, coming back into a squat, with your knees at chest level. Really jump your feet in to give momentum for the jump in the next step.

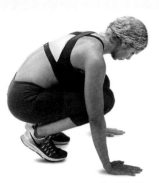

6 Swing your arm straight up and do an explosive jump, getting as much height as you can. This completes one burpee. Repeat for 60 seconds aiming to do a total of 15 burpees.

Sumo squat with bicep curls

The stance for this exercise has to be much wider than for a normal squat.
Focus on squeezing the muscles in your bottom as you stand, as that's
what's going to lift those muscles and help you get the most benefit
from the exercise.

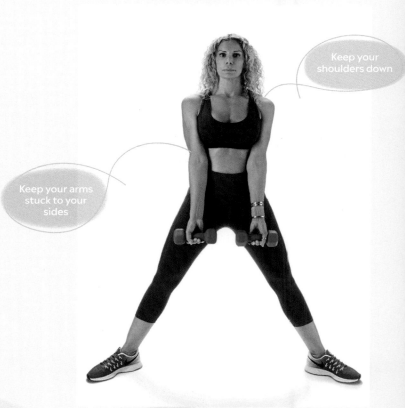

Keep your
shoulders down

Keep your arms
stuck to your
sides

1 Hold a dumbbell in each hand, with your arms
straight down in front of you and palms facing
out. Place your heels not less than 1m (3ft) apart,
with your toes pointing outwards.

WORK

Repeat this exercise for
60 seconds (approximately
15 repetitions).

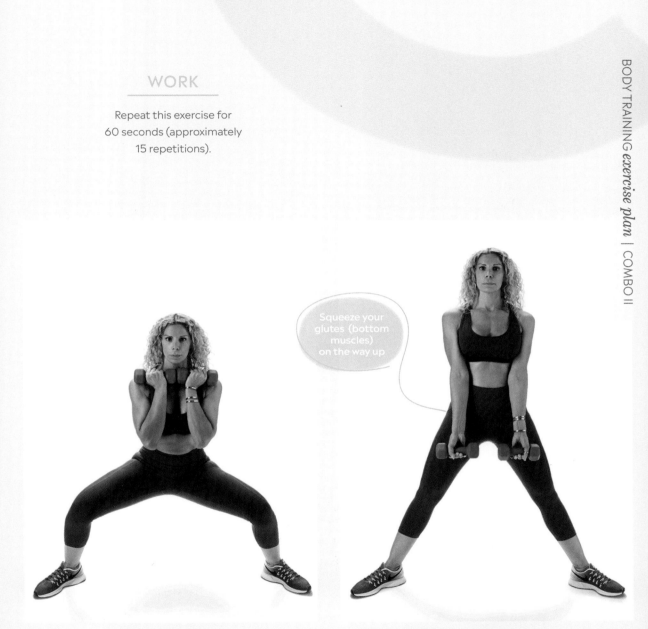

Squeeze your
glutes (bottom
muscles)
on the way up

2 Keeping your weight in your heels and your
shoulders over your hips, bend your knees to
lower your hips. At the same time, bend your elbows
to raise the dumbells to shoulder height.

3 Straighten your legs and arms to return to the
starting position. Squeeze the muscles in your
bottom as you stand. Repeat for 60 seconds.

121

V-sits

Your spine should be in a straight line here, as though you have a thread pulling you straight from the coccyx to the base of your head. Do not hunch your shoulders, use your neck at all, or tuck your chin into your chest. Manage your abilities and choose the right position for you – don't be too ambitious to start with. If you feel your back hurting, change your position until your abs are working instead.

WORK

Repeat this exercise for 60 seconds (approximately 15 repetitions).

Engage your abs

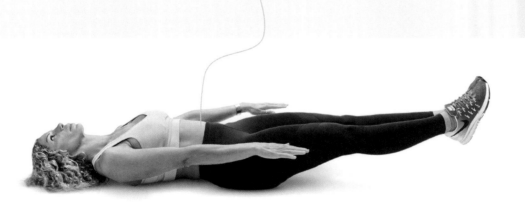

1 Lie on your back with your hands by your sides, then raise your arms off the floor. Engage your abs and lift your legs until they are raised off of the floor.

"If you feel pain in your lower back, don't lean back as far when doing the crunch movement."

- Amélie

Keep your spine elongated

Pull your knees towards your chest

Be careful not to strain your neck

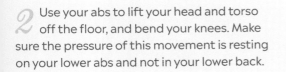

2 Use your abs to lift your head and torso off the floor, and bend your knees. Make sure the pressure of this movement is resting on your lower abs and not in your lower back.

3 Slowly lower your torso while you straighten your legs until your back is on the floor, but your head, shoulders, arms, and legs are raised. Repeat this exercise for 60 seconds.

PHASE TWO *weeks 3–4*

Bent-over row

For this, you should keep your knees and back straight; lean forwards as much as you need to. Hold your arms and elbows close to your sides, squeeze your shoulder blades together, and release down slowly.

WORK

Repeat this exercise for 60 seconds (approximately 15 repetitions).

Lean forwards from the hips

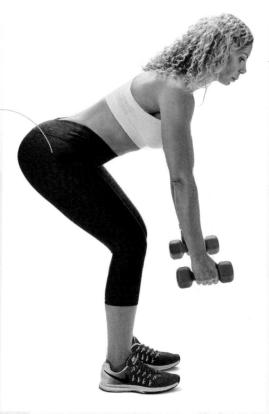

1 Holding a dumbbell in each hand, extend your arms so they are straight. Lean forwards with a straight back. Keep your knees soft and pull your navel towards your spine.

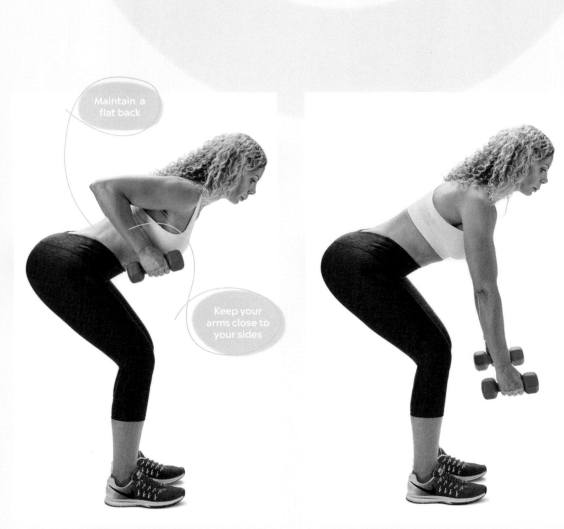

2 Lift the dumbbells straight up to chest level by bending your elbows up behind you, squeezing your shoulder blades together. Keep your elbows in and pointed upwards.

3 Slowly lower the weights back to the starting position. This is one repetition. Repeat Steps 2 and 3 for 60 seconds.

Jump squats

This exercise requires an explosive movement, so form is important. As with any squat, the core muscles aid stability. Landing on your full foot and not your toes is better for your knees. You can also use your arms for momentum.

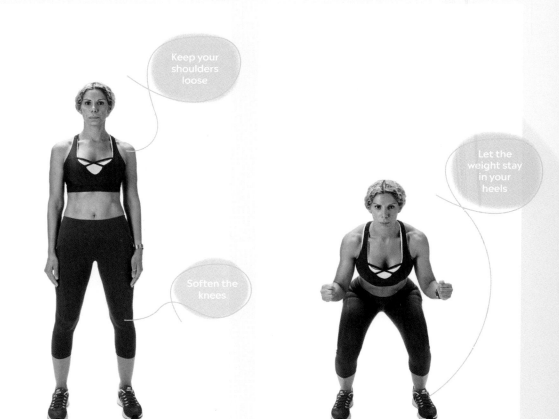

Keep your shoulders loose

Let the weight stay in your heels

Soften the knees

1 Stand with your feet hip-width apart, with your arms by your sides, and your shoulders relaxed.

2 Keeping your weight in your heels, bend your knees, lowering your hips so your thighs are parallel to the floor and your knees no further forwards than your toes.

WORK

Repeat this exercise for
60 seconds (approximately
15 repetitions).

Engage
your lower
abs to jump
higher

Remember to
squat when
you land on
your feet

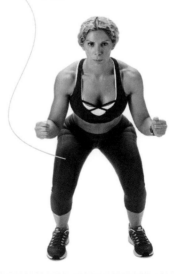

3 Swing your arms to the ceiling as you jump
straight up, pushing off with both feet.

4 Land softly on your full feet, not your
toes, as you return to the squat position.
This is one repetition. Repeat Steps 2–4 for a
total of 60 seconds.

Squat, curl, and press

Take your time here to make sure you break down the movement exactly as spelled out: elbows next to your thighs, bring the dumbbells all the way to your shoulders and – when it comes to the press – do not throw your arms.

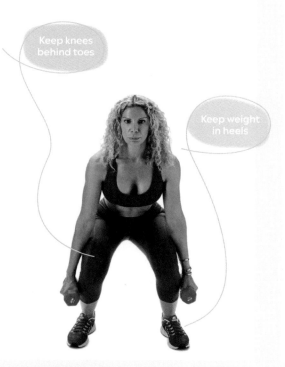

Keep knees behind toes

Keep weight in heels

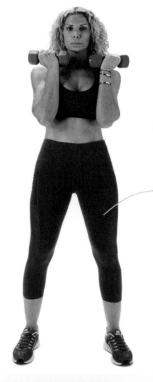

Use your quads (thighs) to drive upwards

1 Stand with your feet hip-width apart. Hold a dumbbell in each hand with your arms by your sides. Bend your knees and lower your hips so your thighs are parallel to the floor.

2 Push through your heels to return to standing. At the same time, bring the weights to your shoulders, palms facing you, performing a biceps curl.

WORK

Repeat this exercise for
60 seconds (approximately
15 repetitions).

*"This is a compound movement,
which engages the entire body.
Form is everything, so don't rush."*

— Amélie

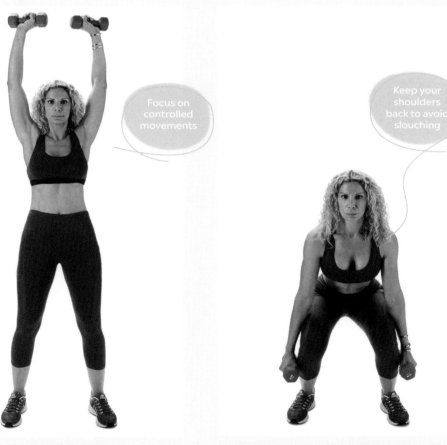

Focus on controlled movements

Keep your shoulders back to avoid slouching

3 With your chest straight ahead, keep your arms moving straight upwards, rotating your forearms so your palms face away from you when your arms are fully extended .

4 Lower your arms back to your sides. Bend your knees and lower your hips to return to the starting position. This is one repetition. Repeat for a total of 60 seconds.

Scissors

You can really feel this exercise work as you're doing it. Take it slowly and make sure that your spine is very firmly on the floor, with your navel pulled into your spine. Keep your neck relaxed and instead focus on the muscles in your core.

WORK

Repeat this exercise for 60 seconds.

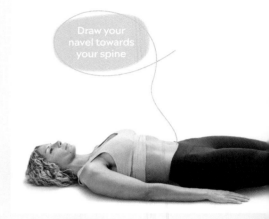

Draw your navel towards your spine

1 Lie on your back with your arms by your sides, palms pressing into the floor. You can place your hands under your bottom if you feel the need to protect your lower back.

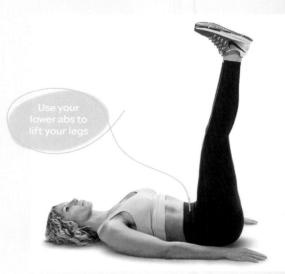

Use your lower abs to lift your legs

2 Bring both legs straight up towards the ceiling, engaging your abdominal muscles and pressing your lower back into the floor.

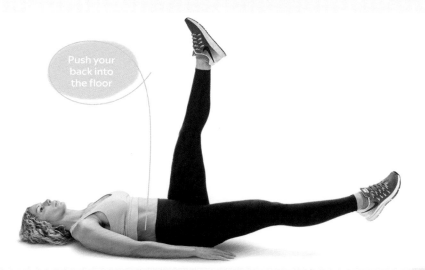

3 Keep your core pulled in and your lower back on the ground. Point your toes and slowly lower your right leg until it's a few centimetres above the floor.

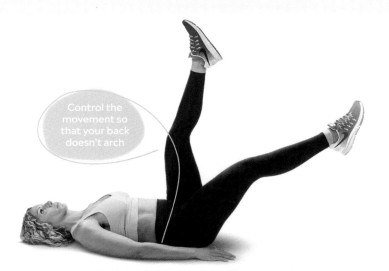

4 "Scissor" your legs, swapping their positions up and down. Keep all the movements controlled. Continue to work for a total of 60 seconds.

Lying chest fly

This is a relatively simple exercise. The key is to make a conscious effort to push your back and feet into the floor. On the outward motion, keep your arms a good 5cm (2in) off the ground, making sure they don't touch it. This way, the pressure is on the chest.

WORK

Repeat this exercise for 60 seconds (approximately 15 repetitions).

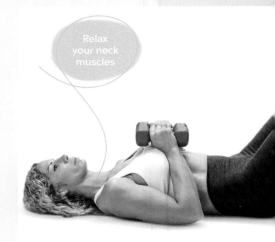

Relax your neck muscles

1 Holding a dumbbell in each hand, lie on your back with your hips and knees both bent and your feet flat on the ground. Press your lower back into the ground.

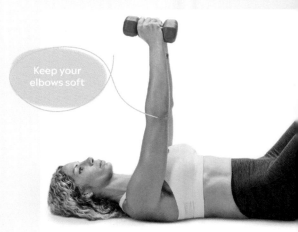

Keep your elbows soft

2 Raise your arms towards the ceiling, palm facing each other, keeping the elbows slig bent and making sure the weights do not touc

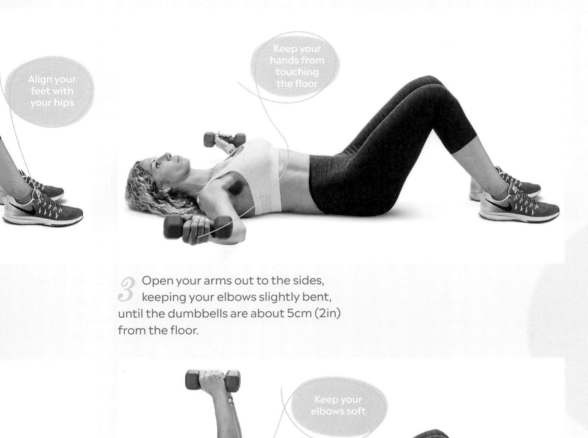

3 Open your arms out to the sides, keeping your elbows slightly bent, until the dumbbells are about 5cm (2in) from the floor.

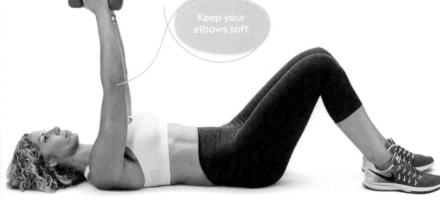

4 Raise your arms back towards the ceiling, bringing the weights together over your chest without them touching. This is one repetition. Repeat steps 2–4 for a total of 60 seconds.

Plank jacks

You should now be familiar with this exercise from Phase One. Remember to keep your core engaged in order to perform it correctly. Don't let your upper body or bottom and hips dip around. To avoid the bouncing, really focus on controlling your movements.

WORK

Repeat this exercise for 60 seconds (approximately 15 repetitions).

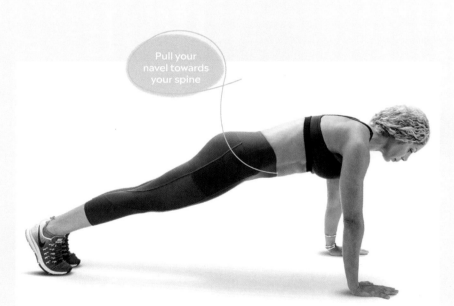

Pull your navel towards your spine

1 Begin in a High plank (see p64), with your body in a straight line, hands placed under your shoulders, and feet together. Don't let your hips drop or your lower back arch.

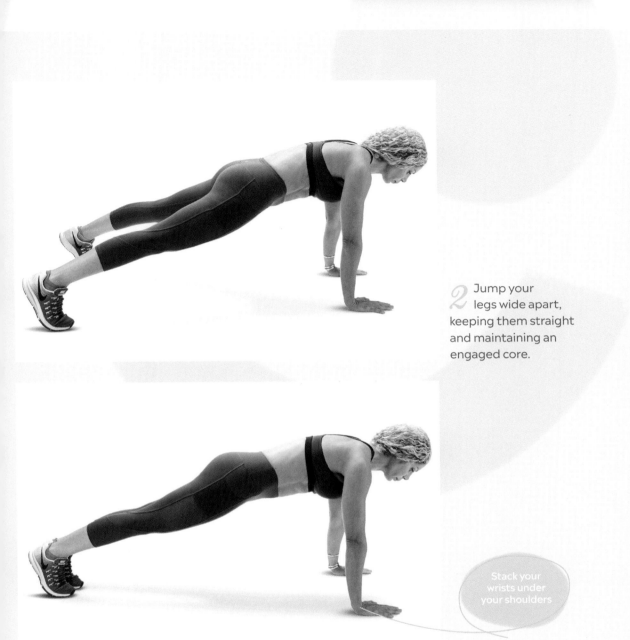

2 Jump your legs wide apart, keeping them straight and maintaining an engaged core.

Stack your wrists under your shoulders

3 Immediately jump your legs back together to return to the starting position. This completes one repetition. Repeat for a total of 60 seconds.

COOL DOWN

Your Cool down should take three minutes: do each of these stretches for 60 seconds with no rests in between.

Happy baby

Happy baby is a soothing hip opener and full-body stretch. You can control the intensity of the stretch with your hands.

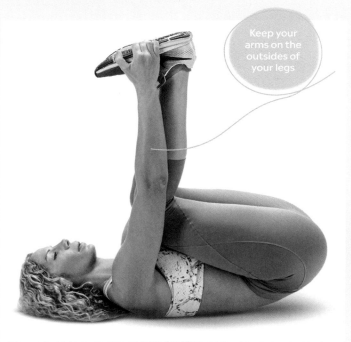

 Keep your arms on the outsides of your legs

1 Lie flat on your back. Bend both knees, and hold the outside edges of your flexed feet with your hands.

2 Gently use your upper-body strengthto press both knees equally towards the floor, below your armpits. Try not to tense your shoulders or chest, but keep everything relaxed.

3 Hold for 60 seconds, taking slow, deep breaths.

Head to knee

This targets the hips and the back of the legs. The stretch you can manage in Head to knee will vary from one session to another, depending on your flexibility. Keep your neck relaxed and focus on your back muscles. If you can't reach your foot, rest your hands on your shin or knee.

WORK

Perform this stretch for 60 seconds.

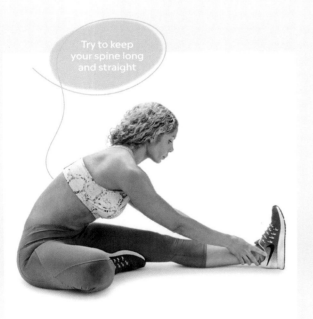

Try to keep your spine long and straight

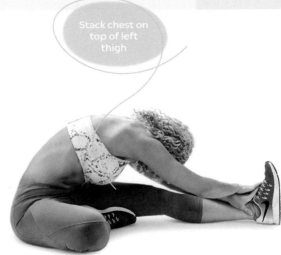

Stack chest on top of left thigh

1 Sit on the ground with your legs out in front of you. Bend your right knee, and place the sole of your right foot against your left inner thigh.

2 Reach both hands towards your left foot. Hold for 30 seconds, relaxing your shoulders away from your ears. Return to sitting, then repeat on the right side.

Triceps stretch

The key to the Triceps stretch is to keep your arm very straight when you bring it next to your ear. Make sure everything is nice and firm, not floppy. Pull your elbow to the point where you can feel a little bit of pleasurable pain in the triceps – it needs some pressure.

WORK

Perform this stretch for 60 seconds.

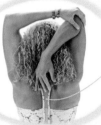

Spread your shoulder blades wide

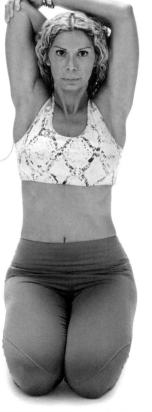

Concentrate on good posture

1 Reach your right arm over your head to lengthen the right side of your body. Maintain the length as you bend your right elbow to bring your fingers to the middle of your upper back

2 Grab your right elbow with your left hand and gently pull the right elbow towards the left-hand side.

3 Increase the stretch, lengthening the right side of your chest even more, by bending sideways to the left.

4 Hold for 15 seconds, then release your arm and return to the starting position. Repeat on the opposite side. Repeat for 60 seconds, alternating sides.

At the beginning, most of the exercises were challenging, but after a couple of weeks what had been harder got easier. It's really gratifying when you start seeing changes.

- Jodie

PHASE *THREE*

weeks 5–6

The goal of Phase Three is to cement what you've put in place over the past four weeks with a PRESERVE EATING PLAN and SUCCESS EXERCISE PLAN. You'll continue to boost the fat-burning process through both your diet and exercise. I'll also give you the relevant mental and physical tools you need to reach your end goal.

PRESERVE
eating plan

During Phase Three you will use the knowledge you acquired over the last four weeks to build your own menu each day. Choose from the lists of breakfast, lunch, dinner, snack, and dessert recipes. The most important thing is learning to balance your meals and make nutritional choices that enhance your weight loss and general wellbeing.

Keep drinking the warm cinnamon water and lemon (see p12) first thing in the morning.

Remember to drink 1.5–2 litres (2¾–3½ pints) of water every day, always take the time to sit down to eat, and finish every day with a mug of herbal tea.

You can pick your breakfast each day, as in Phases One and Two, except for your "Sans Day" (see below). You can also choose to have a smoothie instead of one of the breakfast options.

One day a week you will do a "Sans Day". This means that one day a week you choose to give up either sugar, added fat (butter or oils), carbs (potato, rice, pasta, quinoa), bread (any type), chocolate, or coffee. The aim of the "Sans Day" is to help with fat loss, but also to make you really focus on your diet and food choices.

You can choose to make Jodie's recipes (see pp168–71) one day a week instead of repeating recipes from earlier in the week.

You will need a steamer, non-stick frying pan, blender, wok, and kitchen scales to hand.

BREAKFASTS

CHOOSE ONE FROM THE BREAKFAST OPTIONS, OR HAVE A SMOOTHIE
(pp146–47 or 148)

Weeks 5–6

SMOOTHIES	LUNCHES	DINNERS	DESSERTS
GREEN SMOOTHIE (p148)	STRAWBERRY AND BABY SPINACH SALAD (p150)	STEAK STIR-FRY (p160)	1 5 LEVEL TBSP FULL-FAT PLAIN YOGURT, SWEETENED WITH 1 TSP AGAVE SYRUP
APPLE SMOOTHIE (p148)	SALMON, SWEET POTATO, AND BROCCOLI (p152)	KIWI SALMON (p160)	2 1 APPLE
AVOCADO SMOOTHIE (p148)	PENNE AND FETA SALAD (p152)	CREAMY STEAK AND SWEET POTATO CHIPS (p162)	3 1 BANANA
VIOLET SMOOTHIE (p148)	AVOCADO CASSE-CROÛTE (p155)	LAMB KOFTA WITH SPICED QUINOA (p164)	4 SMALL BOWL OF BERRIES
	SMOKED SALMON, RICE, AND LENTIL SALAD (p155)	SPICY BOMBAY TURKEY (p164)	
	QUINOA AND BROCCOLI SALAD (p156)	EXPRESS SPAG BOL (p166)	
	ALMOND AND TOFU STIR-FRY (p156)	CANCUN TOMATO (p166)	

"Sans Day"

One day a week give up either sugar, added fat (butter or oils), carbs (potato, rice, pasta, quinoa), bread (any type), chocolate, or coffee. Each recipe in this phase is appropriately labelled.

PRESERVE
weekly shopping list

During Phase Three you will build your own meal plan rather than following a set plan each day. Below is a shopping list for if you eat each lunch and dinner option once, but you can choose to create a different plan if you prefer. As in the previous two phases, breakfasts and snacks are your choice, and you can also choose to mix in Jodie's recipes one day a week. In this phase, snacks are also your choice (see p143). Shop accordingly.

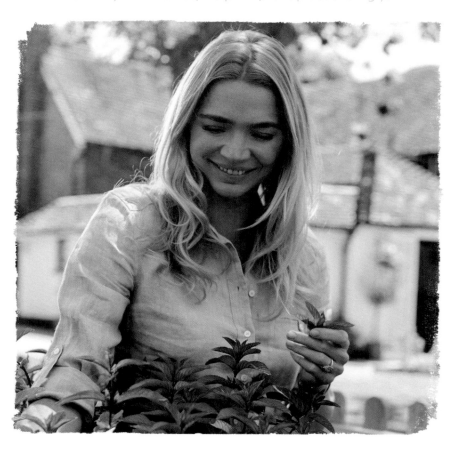

Fruits and vegetables

Avocado 1

Broccoli unlimited

Carrots 2

Celery 2 sticks

Garlic 18 cloves
or about 3 heads

Ginger, fresh root
about 1 large thumb

Green beans, extra-fine
100g (3½oz)

Herbs
Buy your herbs in
bunches or packs.
You will need:
Basil
Coriander
Mint
Oregano
Thyme leaves

Lemons 2

Lettuce
unlimited Romaine,
iceberg, rocket

Lime 1

Kiwi fruit 1

Mushrooms, shiitake
75g (2½oz)

Onions 4

Pak choi 2 heads

Peppers, red 1

Shallots 2

Spinach 400g (14oz),
or more if you like

Spring onions 4

Strawberries 10

Sweet potatoes 3

Tomatoes, regular 3

Tomato, beef
1 (the large type, for
stuffing)

Tomatoes, cherry
13 (about 1 punnet)

Meat, fish, soya, and eggs

Beef, minced (lean)
100g (3½oz)

Chicken breast, raw,
free-range
1 x 140g (5oz)

Lamb, minced
150g (5½oz)

Salmon fillet, wild
2 x 200g (7oz) each

Salmon, smoked
3 slices

Steak, sirloin
2 x 200g (7oz) each

Tofu, smoked
125g (4½oz)

Turkey, minced, free-
range
100g (3½oz)

Dairy and non-dairy alternatives

Cheese, feta
50g (1¾oz)

Cheese, Parmesan
30g (1oz)

Cream cheese, or
non-dairy alternative,
full-fat
1 tsp

Crème fraîche, half-fat
1 tbsp

Store cupboard

You'll still need some
of the supplies you
bought for Phases One
and Two, so keep track of
what you might be
running low on.

Almonds

Bay leaves, dried

Bread, wholemeal,
sourdough, or rye

Chicken stock, organic

Chickpeas, canned

Chilli powder

Cinnamon, ground

Coriander, ground

Cumin, ground

Cumin seeds

Curry paste

Curry powder

Dark agave syrup

Extra virgin organic
olive oil

Extra virgin olive
oil spray

Greaseproof paper

Herbes de Provence

Lentils, Puy

Mustard, Dijon

Oil, coconut

Oil, sesame

Olives, black

Pasta, wholegrain penne
and wholewheat
spaghetti

Quinoa

Rice, brown

Soy sauce,
reduced salt

Tomatoes, canned
chopped

Vinegar, organic apple
cider

Walnuts

Beverage

Herbal tea
Any of your choice

Water, sparkling
or still
You can choose either,
as long as every day you
drink 1.5–2 litres (2¾–3½
pints).

Breakfasts, snacks,
desserts, and herbal teas
are all your choice. Look
through the recipes
(pp142–71), decide what
you'd like to eat, and then
shop accordingly.

BREAKFASTS
and SNACKS

Eat any of these breakfasts each morning during Weeks 5–6, but don't forget to incorporate a "Sans Day" (see p142–43) one day a week. If you are hungry after lunch, have one of these snacks in the afternoon, again, taking in to account your "Sans Day" requirements.

Breakfast options

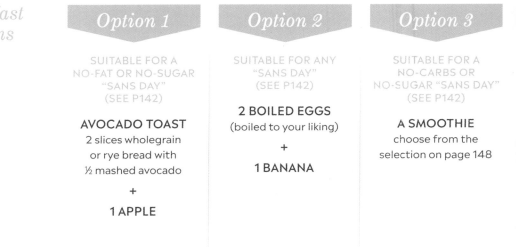

Option 1

SUITABLE FOR A
NO-FAT OR NO-SUGAR
"SANS DAY"
(SEE P142)

AVOCADO TOAST
2 slices wholegrain
or rye bread with
½ mashed avocado

+

1 APPLE

Option 2

SUITABLE FOR ANY
"SANS DAY"
(SEE P142)

2 BOILED EGGS
(boiled to your liking)

+

1 BANANA

Option 3

SUITABLE FOR A
NO-CARBS OR
NO-SUGAR "SANS DAY"
(SEE P142)

A SMOOTHIE
choose from the
selection on page 148

Snack options
Choose any one of these snacks to eat in the afternoon to bridge the gap between lunch and dinner.

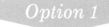

Option 1

**1 BANANA AND
5 PRUNES**

Option 2

**1 APPLE AND
10 ALMONDS**

Option 3

**1 SLICE WHOLEMEAL
SOURDOUGH
BREAD AND
3 DRIED APRICOTS**

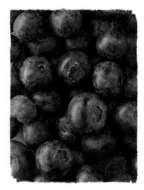

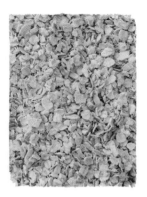

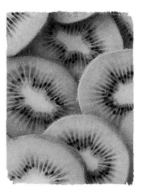

Option 4

SUITABLE FOR A
NO-SUGAR "SANS DAY"
(SEE P142)

**EGG WHITE AND
SPINACH OMELETTE**
Make as on page 89,
adding a handful of baby
spinach to the egg whites
as they cook.

+

**1 SLICE WHOLEMEAL
SOURDOUGH OR
RYE BREAD**

Option 5

SUITABLE FOR A NO-FAT
"SANS DAY" (SEE P142)

**OVERNIGHT
PORRIDGE WITH
ALMONDS**
Prepare this the night
before. Half-fill a small
bowl or a mug with rolled
oats and just cover with
boiling water. Stir, cover,
and chill overnight in the
fridge. In the morning,
add 5–6 almonds and
1 tbsp agave syrup. Spoon
into a small saucepan and
placeover a medium heat.
Bring to the boil, stirring,
until thickened.

Option 6

SUITABLE FOR ANY
"SANS DAY"
(SEE P142)

**ALMOND SOYA
YOGURT BOWL**
Mix 4 tbsp almond soya
yogurt with 1 tsp almond
butter and a handful of
blueberries, strawberries,
or pomegranate seeds.

Option 7

SUITABLE FOR A
NO-SUGAR "SANS DAY"
(SEE P142)

**WHOLEMEAL
SOURDOUGH OR
RYE BREAD**
1 slice with a thin
layer of butter

+

SMOKED SALMON

+

**BLUEBERRIES OR
STRAWBERRIES**
small side dish

Option 4

**5 LEVEL TBSP SOYA
YOGURT AND
½ GRAPEFRUIT**

Option 5

**ALMOND BANANA
SMOOTHIE**
Blend 1 banana with
200ml (7fl oz) almond
milk

Option 6

**1 KIWI FRUIT AND
2 SQUARES OF
70 PER CENT DARK
CHOCOLATE**

Option 7

**2 OATCAKES WITH
ALMOND BUTTER**

SMOOTHIES

For all the smoothies here, just rinse the fruit and vegetables, whizz them in a blender with all the other ingredients, then drink up! Each has a high concentration of essential nutrients packed into one enjoyable drink.

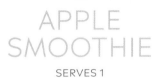

Option 1

GREEN SMOOTHIE

SERVES 1

1 apple, cored and chopped
1 celery stick, chopped
handful of spinach
2 slices of fresh root ginger, peeled
pinch of ground cinnamon

Option 2

APPLE SMOOTHIE

SERVES 1

1 apple, cored and chopped
1 mug of spinach
1 mug of kale
1 tbsp Greek yogurt
3–4 ice cubes

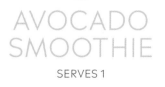

Option 3

AVOCADO SMOOTHIE

SERVES 1

½ avocado, peeled and pitted
1 apple, cored and chopped
1 tsp dark agave syrup
3–4 ice cubes

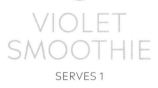

Option 4

VIOLET SMOOTHIE

SERVES 1

2 handfuls of blueberries
1 tbsp soya yogurt
250ml (9fl oz) almond milk
a few mint leaves
3–4 ice cubes

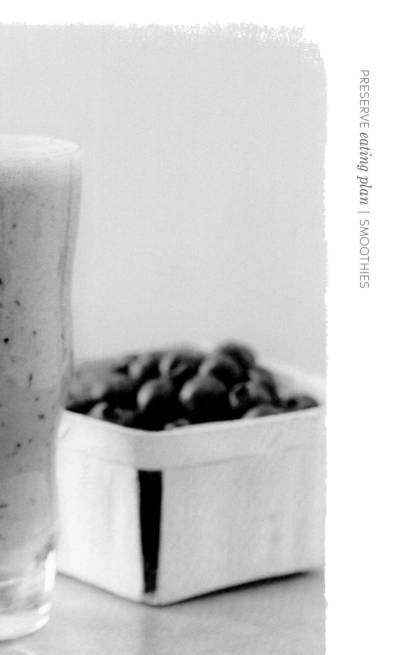

Violet smoothie

LUNCHES

Pick and choose from the following 7 lunch options (see pp150–56), taking in to account that one day a week you will need to do a "Sans Day" (see p142-43).

Option 1

STRAWBERRY AND BABY SPINACH SALAD

SUITABLE FOR A NO-CARBS "SANS DAY" (SEE P142)

SERVES 1

3 cups of baby leaf spinach (or more if you are hungry)

10 strawberries, hulled and halved

3 cherry tomatoes, halved

2 tbsp cooked chickpeas

For the dressing

½ tsp Dijon mustard

½ tsp apple cider vinegar

1 tsp extra virgin olive oil

salt and pepper

1 In a large serving bowl, mix together the spinach, strawberries, tomatoes, and chickpeas, and set aside.

2 In a small bowl or a cup, whisk together the mustard, cider vinegar, and olive oil. Season to taste with salt and pepper.

3 Drizzle the salad with the dressing and gently toss to coat.

Dessert

Choose a dessert from the list on page 143

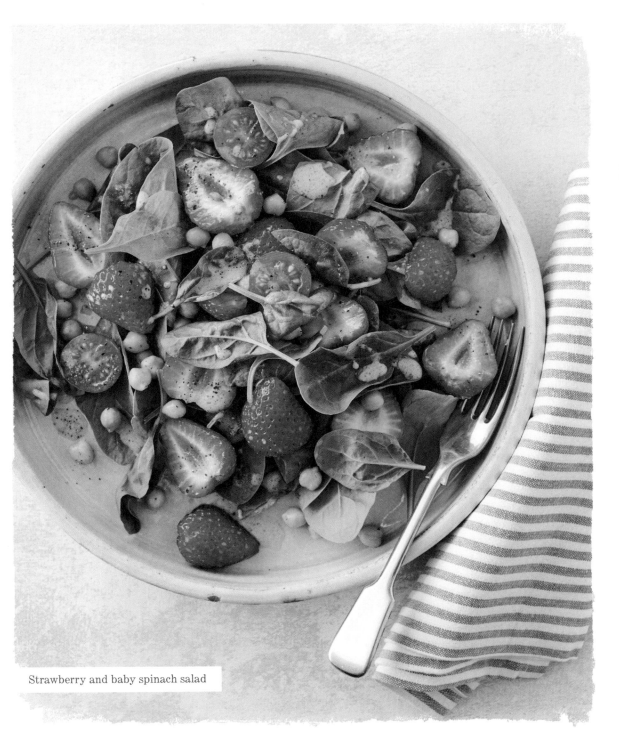

Strawberry and baby spinach salad

SALMON, SWEET POTATO, AND BROCCOLI

**SUITABLE FOR A NO-FAT "SANS DAY"
(SEE P142)**

SERVES 1

1 small sweet potato	small bowl of broccoli florets
salt and pepper	
1 wild salmon fillet, about 200g (7oz)	

1 Cube and steam the sweet potato for 20 minutes. Alternatively, bake whole, wrapped in foil, in a 180°C (350°F/Gas 4) oven for about 30 minutes, or until a sharp knife pierces it easily. Mash the sweet potato and season to taste with salt and pepper.

2 Meanwhile, either grill the salmon fillet for 5 minutes, without turning, or fry it in a dry non-stick frying pan over a medium-high heat, turning once, for 2–3 minutes each side.

3 At the same time, steam the broccoli for about 5 minutes.

4 Serve the salmon with the mashed sweet potato and steamed broccoli.

Dessert

Choose a dessert from the list on page 143

PENNE AND FETA SALAD

**SUITABLE FOR A NO-SUGAR "SANS DAY"
(SEE P142)**

SERVES 1

100g (3½oz) wholegrain penne	handful of basil leaves
salt and pepper	4 cherry tomatoes, halved
50g (1¾oz) feta cheese, crumbled	**For the dressing**
	juice of ½ lemon
6 black olives, pitted	1 tsp extra virgin olive oil

1 Cook the pasta in salted boiling water according to the packet instructions. Rinse under cold running water, drain well, and let cool.

2 In a large serving bowl, mix together the feta, olives, basil, and tomatoes. Add the cooled pasta and carefully stir it with the other ingredients, then set aside.

3 In a small bowl or a cup, whisk together the lemon juice and olive oil until the dressing is thoroughly mixed. Season to taste with salt and pepper.

4 Drizzle the salad with the dressing and gently toss to coat.

Dessert

Choose a dessert from the list on page 143

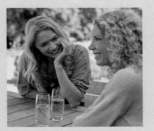

Jodie & Amélie

"

Amélie

You're in the final phase of my plan now. How has it made a difference to your body?

Jodie

I've always been quite physical and done lots of exercise, but the middle area of my body needed addressing. For me it wasn't so much about getting thin, but I'm more toned now. I've bought a smaller pair of jeans.

"

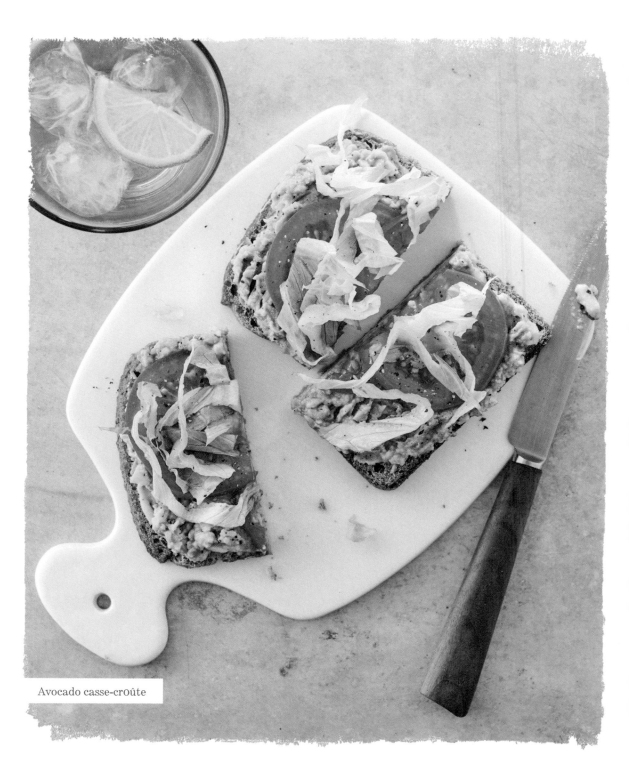

Avocado casse-croûte

Option 4

AVOCADO CASSE-CROÛTE

**SUITABLE FOR A NO-SUGAR "SANS DAY"
(SEE P142)**

SERVES 1

½ avocado

1 tsp Dijon mustard

2 slices rye or wholemeal
sourdough bread

salt and pepper

1 tomato, sliced

handful of Romaine
lettuce, shredded

1 Mash the avocado in a bowl. Spread the mustard onto the bread, then the mashed avocado.

2 Season to taste with salt and pepper, then place the tomato slice on top and scatter over the lettuce.

3 Cut the slices in half to serve.

Dessert

Choose a dessert from the
list on page 143

Option 5

SMOKED SALMON, RICE, AND LENTIL SALAD

**SUITABLE FOR A NO-SUGAR "SANS DAY"
(SEE P142)**

SERVES 1

100g (3½oz) brown rice

3 slices of smoked salmon,
shredded

100g (3½oz) cooked Puy
lentils

1 spring onion, finely
chopped

1 tbsp crushed walnuts

For the dressing

juice of 1 lime

pinch of cumin

salt and pepper

1 Cook the rice according to the packet instructions, then drain and allow to cool.

2 In a large serving bowl, mix the cooled rice with the salmon, lentils, spring onion, and walnuts.

3 In a small bowl or a cup, whisk together the lime juice and cumin and season well with salt and pepper.

4 Drizzle the salad with the dressing, stir gently, and serve.

Dessert

Choose a dessert from the
list on page 143

QUINOA AND BROCCOLI SALAD

**SUITABLE FOR A NO-FAT "SANS DAY"
(SEE P142)**

SERVES 1

100g (3½oz) quinoa

1 mug of broccoli florets

2 spring onions, finely chopped

6 cherry tomatoes, halved

For the dressing

½ tsp Dijon mustard

1 garlic clove, crushed

1 tbsp apple cider vinegar

salt and pepper

1   Cook the quinoa according to the packet instructions. Drain if necessary, then set aside to cool slightly.

2   Meanwhile, steam the broccoli until just tender, but do not overcook it.

3   In a large serving bowl, mix together the quinoa, broccoli, spring onions, and tomatoes.

4   In a small bowl or a cup, whisk together the dressing ingredients with a fork. Season to taste with salt and pepper.

5   Pour the dressing over the salad and stir gently to coat.

Dessert

Choose a dessert from the
list on page 143

ALMOND AND TOFU STIR-FRY

**SUITABLE FOR A NO-CARB "SANS DAY"
(SEE P142)**

SERVES 1

1 tsp sesame oil

1 garlic clove, crushed

1 tbsp finely grated root ginger

125g (4½oz) smoked tofu, chopped

½ red pepper, sliced

2 spring onions, finely sliced

100g (3½oz) extra-fine green beans

1 tbsp reduced salt soy sauce

2 level tbsp chopped almonds

1   Add the sesame oil to a wok and place over a high heat. Leave for 1½ minutes to get very hot.

2   Add the garlic, ginger, tofu, red pepper, spring onions, and green beans to the wok and stir-fry for just under 1 minute.

3   Stir in the soy sauce and almonds and serve immediately.

Dessert

Choose a dessert from the
list on page 143

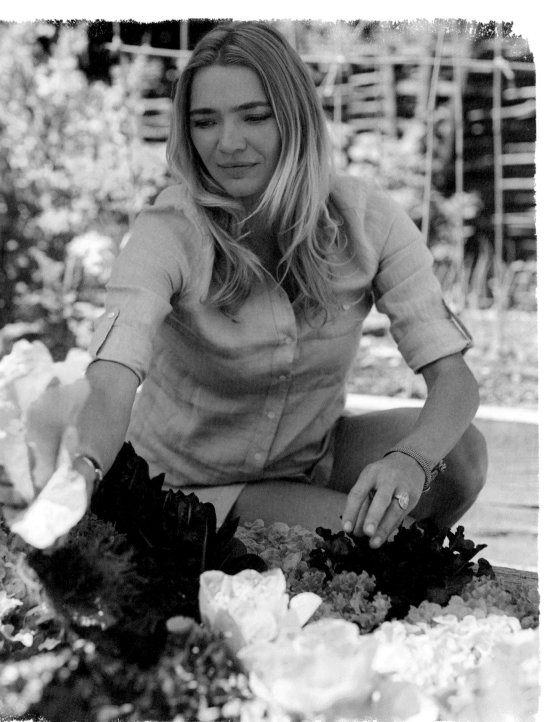

When I need to re-centre I go for a walk and say my thank yous. I list everything I am grateful for, and it helps me put everything in perspective.

- Jodie

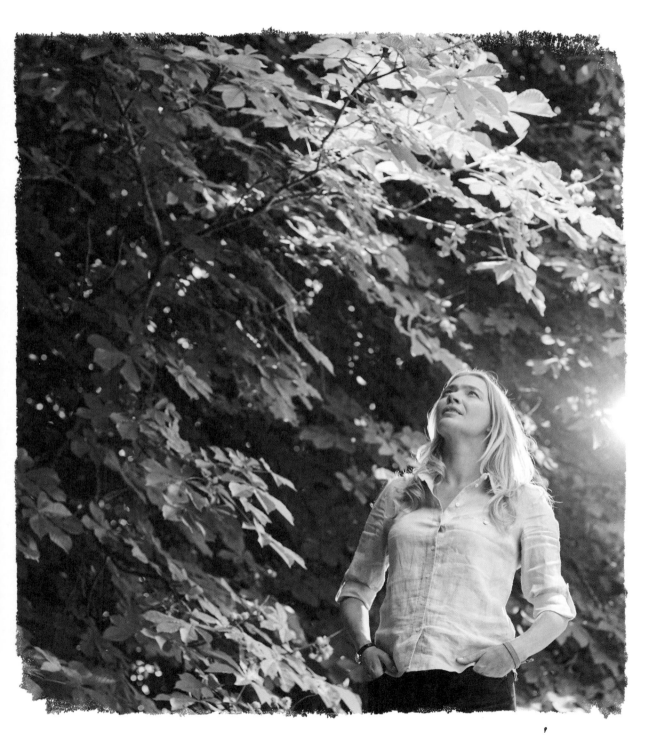

DINNERS

In the first two phases you should have acquired new habits to keep you healthy and burning fat. Stick to them now; choose only wholegrain carbs and eat vegetables with every dish.

Option 1

STEAK STIR-FRY

SUITABLE FOR A NO-CARB "SANS DAY" (SEE P142)

SERVES 1

100g (3½oz) extra-fine green beans

2 tbsp sesame oil

1 sirloin steak, about 200g (7oz) sliced

1 onion, sliced

2 garlic cloves, crushed

½ tsp finely grated root ginger

1 carrot, sliced

75g (2½oz) shiitake mushrooms, sliced

¼ red pepper, sliced

3 tbsp soy sauce

2 heads of pak choi, quartered lengthways

½ head of broccoli, cut into small florets

juice of 1 lemon

cooked brown rice, to serve (if not a "Sans Day")

salt and pepper

1 Boil the green beans for 5 minutes. Drain and set aside.

2 Heat 1 tbsp of the oil in a wok over a high heat. When it's smoking, add the steak and stir-fry until brown. Remove from the wok and set aside.

3 Add the remaining oil to the wok. When smoking, add the onion, garlic, and ginger. Stir-fry for 1 minute, then add the carrot, mushrooms, and pepper. Stir-fry for 3 minutes then stir in 2 tablespoons of water and the soy sauce. Add the pak choi and broccoli andstir-fry for 2 minutes.

5 Return the steak along with the green beans to the wok, stir-fry for 1 minute, then serve with the brown rice.

Dessert

Choose a dessert from the list on page 143

Option 2

KIWI SALMON

SUITABLE FOR A NO-FAT OR NO-SUGAR "SANS DAY" (SEE P142)

SERVES 1

1 sweet potato

1 salmon fillet, about 200g (7oz)

salt and pepper

steamed spinach, to serve

For the salsa

1 kiwi fruit, peeled and finely chopped

1 spring onion, finely chopped

½ avocado, peeled, pitted, and chopped

2 tbsp chopped coriander

1 tbsp lime juice

1 Preheat the oven to 180°C (350°F/Gas 4). Wrap the sweet potato in foil and bake for about 30 minutes, or until a sharp knife pierces it easily with no resistance.

2 Meanwhile, line a baking tray with greaseproof paper and place the salmon on top. Season with salt and pepper, and cook in the oven for 10 minutes.

3 Mix all the ingredients for the salsa together in a bowl. Season to taste with salt and pepper.

4 Serve the salmon with the salsa spooned on top, with the sweet potato and steamed spinach on the side.

Dessert

Choose a dessert from the list on page 143

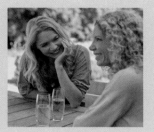

Jodie&Amélie

66 *Amélie*
Have you had any cravings?

Jodie
I've found it easy to take things one day at a time.
One day without coffee, or chocolate, or a certain
food is manageable. I used to have perhaps two
cups of coffee a day, but I've completely fallen in
love with the lemon and cinnamon drink. If I have
a cup of coffee now, my body feels it. I'm being
kinder to myself and drinking your warm water
with lemon and cinnamon instead.

Amélie
The cinnamon is a powerful anti-
inflammatory, lemon juice helps to
clean the liver, and the warm water
helps you feel full. 99

CREAMY STEAK AND SWEET POTATO CHIPS

SUITABLE FOR A NO-SUGAR "SANS DAY" (SEE P142)

SERVES 1

1 sweet potato

olive oil spray

salt and pepper

1 tbsp extra virgin olive oil

1 shallot, sliced

1 garlic clove, crushed

1 tsp herbes de Provence

1 tbsp half-fat crème fraîche

1 sirloin steak, about 200g (7oz)

steamed spinach, to serve

1 Preheat the oven to 200°C (400°F/Gas 6) and line a baking tray with greaseproof paper. Peel the sweet potato and cut it into thick chips. Arrange them on the prepared tray, lightly coat them with the olive oil spray, and season with salt and pepper. Place in the oven and cook for about 20 minutes.

2 Meanwhile, place ½ tbsp of the olive oil in a saucepan over a medium heat and add the shallot. Fry until soft, stirring often. Add the garlic and herbes de Provence. Leave to cook for 1 minute, then stir in the crème fraîche. Season to taste and set aside.

3 Place a frying pan over a high heat and add the remaining olive oil. Season the steak with salt and pepper, add to the hot pan, and cook to your liking.

4 Serve the steak with the sauce on top, alongside the sweet potato chips and steamed spinach.

Dessert

Choose a dessert from the list on page 143

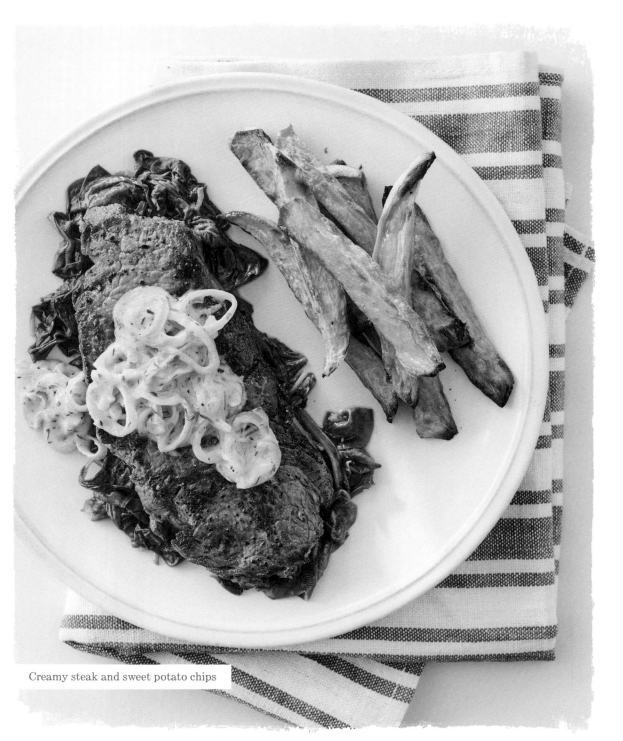

Creamy steak and sweet potato chips

Option 4

LAMB KOFTA WITH SPICED QUINOA

SUITABLE FOR A NO-SUGAR "SANS DAY" (SEE P142)

SERVES 1

For the kofta

150g (5½oz) lean minced lamb
½ onion, finely chopped or grated
1 tbsp chopped coriander
1 tbsp chopped mint leaves
½ tsp ground coriander
¼ tsp chilli powder
salt and pepper
1 tbsp extra virgin olive oil

For the quinoa

100g (3½oz) quinoa
1 tsp extra virgin olive oil
1 garlic clove, crushed
½ tsp ground cinnamon
½ tsp chilli powder
1 tsp cumin seeds
½ tsp ground coriander
½ tsp coconut oil

1 Start with the kofta. In a bowl, mix the lamb, onion, coriander, mint, and ground spices, and season with salt and pepper.

2 Roll the meat into kofta shapes and leave to chill in the fridge for 30 minutes.

3 Meanwhile, prepare the quinoa according to the packet instructions. Drain, then fluff it up with a fork.

4 To finish the quinoa, heat the olive oil in a frying pan and fry the garlic for 1 minute, then add all the spices and cook for a further minute. Remove from the heat.

5 Add the quinoa to the frying pan, along with the coconut oil. Stir to coat all the grains in the oil and spice mixture and set aside.

6 To cook the kofta, preheat a frying pan over a medium-high heat for 30 seconds, then add the olive oil. Brown the kofta on all sides until cooked through.

7 Serve the kofta with the quinoa.

Dessert

Choose a dessert from the list on page 143

Option 5

SPICY BOMBAY TURKEY

SUITABLE FOR A NO-CARB "SANS DAY" (SEE P142)

SERVES 1

1 tbsp olive oil
1 onion, finely chopped
1 garlic clove, crushed
100g (3½oz) free-range minced turkey
1 tbsp curry paste
100ml (3½fl oz) chicken stock

100g (3½oz) canned chopped tomatoes
100g (3½oz) canned chickpeas, rinsed and drained
handful of spinach
cooked brown rice, to serve (if not a "Sans Day")

1 Place the olive oil in a saucepan over a medium-low heat. Add the onion and fry gently for 5–6 minutes.

2 Increase the heat to medium, add the garlic and the minced turkey, and cook for 5 minutes. Stir in the curry paste and leave to fry for another minute.

3 Add the stock, tomatoes, and chickpeas, and stir the mixture together. Bring to the boil, then reduce the heat and partially cover with the lid. Cook for 15–20 minutes, until the sauce has reduced and thickened.

4 Add the spinach and cook for another 2 minutes. Serve with wholegrain rice.

Dessert

Choose a dessert from the list on page 143

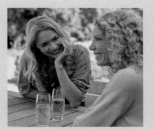

Jodie & Amélie

" Jodie

Do you have any advice for people when they eat out? Are there any good options?

Amélie

At an Italian restaurant, go for a pizza Margherita or tomato-based pasta. At a Japanese restaurant, forgo the sushi and choose sashimi, salad, and miso soup instead. When going for curry, choose tandoori baked dishes and not breads. At the pub, roast chicken salads (dressing on the side), steak, and veggies are all good options. If dessert is a cake (it often is), ask if there is fruit instead. "

" Jodie

And what about if you're travelling?

Amélie

If you're on a plane, have a protein bar in your handbag and avoid the snacks they give out. If you're at a hotel and need breakfast, have yogurt and fruit. At other meals, have meat and veggies. "

EXPRESS SPAG BOL

**SUITABLE FOR A SUGAR-FREE "SANS DAY"
(SEE P142)**

SERVES 1

1 tbsp extra virgin
olive oil

1 onion, finely chopped

100g (3½oz)
lean minced beef

2 garlic cloves, crushed

2 tomatoes, peeled and
finely chopped

1 carrot, finely chopped

1 celery stick, finely sliced

1 bay leaf

½ tsp thyme leaves

salt and pepper

100g (3½oz) wholewheat
spaghetti

30g (1oz) Parmesan
cheese, finely grated

1 In a saucepan, heat up the olive oil over a medium heat, then add the onion, the beef, and the garlic. Cook, stirring, until the beef has browned and the onion has started to soften.

2 Add the tomatoes, carrot, and celery, then stir in the bay leaf and thyme. Season to taste with salt and pepper, leave to simmer for 10 minutes, then remove the bay leaf.

3 Meanwhile, cook the spaghetti until al dente (this is usually about 1 minute less than the time suggested on the packet), then drain.

4 Place the spaghetti in a wide serving bowl and ladle the sauce on top. Sprinkle over the Parmesan and serve.

Dessert

Choose a dessert from the
list on page 143

CANCUN TOMATO

**SUITABLE FOR A NO-CARB "SANS DAY"
(SEE P142)**

SERVES 1

½ tbsp extra virgin
olive oil

1 free-range chicken
breast, about 140g (5oz)

1 beef tomato

1 tsp full-fat cream
cheese, or non-dairy
alternative

¼ tsp oregano

1 shallot, finely chopped

salt and pepper

100g (3½oz) cooked
quinoa, to serve (if not a
"Sans Day")

1 Preheat the oven to 180°C (350°F/Gas 4) and line a baking tray with greaseproof paper. Place a frying pan over a medium heat and add the olive oil. When it is hot add the chicken and cook for 10–12 minutes, or until it is no longer pink on the inside when sliced. Remove from the heat and set aside.

2 Hollow out the tomato, but reserve both the flesh and the tomato. When the chicken breast is cool enough to handle, chop it finely.

3 Mix the reserved tomato flesh with the cooked chicken, cream cheese, oregano, and shallot. Season to taste with salt and pepper.

4 Using a teaspoon, carefully stuff the mixture back into the hollowed-out tomato and place on the prepared tray. Roast in the oven for 15–20 minutes. Serve with a side of quinoa (if you're not on a "Sans Day").

Dessert

Choose a dessert from the
list on page 143

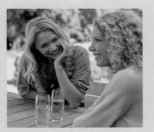

Jodie & Amélie

"

Amélie
Have you found the six weeks
too much?

Jodie
Doing a longer programme definitely
helps. It becomes more of a habit, you
retrain your brain. I can read my body
better now. Those quick-fix diet and
exercise plans are not enough. "

Jodie's recipe

CREAM OF COURGETTE SOUP

Sweetly satisfying, with protein from the nuts to keep you feeling full, this is so easy to make. It's also a great way to use up a chicken carcass left over from a roast. You can omit the chicken and substitute 600ml vegetable stock to make it a vegetarian dish.

PREP 15 MINS
COOK 60–90 MINS
SERVES 2–3

leftover whole chicken carcass

1 tbsp extra virgin olive oil

1 carrot, roughly chopped

1 large onion, roughly chopped

1 stick of celery, chopped

2 garlic cloves, peeled and halved

salt and pepper

3 medium courgettes, roughly chopped (400g/14oz)

120ml (4fl oz) single cream

salt and pepper

toasted flaked almonds, to garnish

1 Put the chicken carcass into a stockpot over a medium heat. Add 750ml (1¼ pints) water, or enough to cover the carcass. Leave to simmer gently, uncovered, for 30 minutes to an hour.

2 Remove the stockpot from the heat and leave to cool slightly. Then strain the stock into a large heatproof bowl. Discard the carcass and set the stock aside.

3 When the stock is ready, add the olive oil to a large saucepan over a medium heat. When hot, add the carrot, onion, celery, and garlic. Give them a stir, season with salt and pepper, and cover with the lid. Leave the mixture to sweat for 5 minutes. Now stir in the chopped courgettes and leave to sweat for a further 5 minutes, covered.

4 Remove the lid and add the chicken stock. Bring to a simmer and leave to cook for 20 minutes, partially covered. Remove the soup from the heat and leave to cool slightly. Then add to a blender and whizz until smooth. Return the soup to the saucepan over a medium-low heat.

5 Stir the cream into the soup and season to taste with salt and pepper. Gently re-heat, but do not allow it to boil.

6 To serve, divide the soup between serving bowls, and garnish with a few toasted flaked almonds.

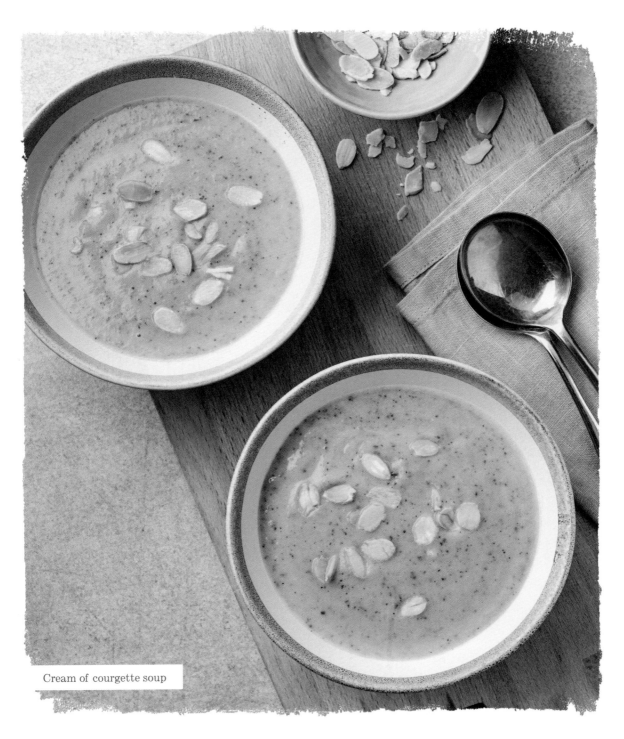

Cream of courgette soup

Jodie's recipe

SHEPHERD'S PIE

Shepherd's pie –everyone's favourite - with the carbs dialled right down. The whole family will love eating this deeply comforting dish. To finish, a quick flash under a hot grill browns the topping.

PREP 15 MINS
COOK 60-65 MINS, PLUS RESTING
SERVES 4

---

1 tbsp rapeseed oil

1 large onion, finely chopped

2 medium carrots, chopped

500g (1lb 2oz) lamb mince

2 tbsp tomato purée

generous splash of Worcestershire sauce

salt and pepper

400ml (14fl oz) beef or lamb stock

900g (2lb) sweet potatoes, peeled and diced

15g (½oz) butter

salt and pepper

1. Place the oil in a medium saucepan over a low heat. Add the onion and carrots, give them a stir, and leave to soften for 3-4 minutes. Turn the heat to medium and crumble in the lamb mince. Brown the meat, tipping off any fat it releases as it cooks. Stir in the tomato purée and Worcestershire sauce, and season with salt and pepper. Leave to cook for 3-4 minutes then pour over the stock, stir, and bring to a simmer. Cover and leave to cook for 40 minutes, removing the lid after 20 minutes.

2. Meanwhile, make the sweet potato mash. Boil the potatoes in a saucepan of salted water over a high heat for 10-15 minutes until tender. Drain, then mash with the butter.

3. Preheat the oven to 200°C (400°F/Gas 6). Place the mince in an ovenproof dish, top with the mash, and ruffle the surface with a fork*. Bake for 20-25 minutes, until the top is starting to colour and the mince mixture is bubbling through at the edges. Leave to rest for 5 minutes before serving

*The pie can now be chilled and frozen for up to a month. To bake from frozen, cook at 160°C (325°F/ Gas 3) for 60 minutes to 1 hour 20 minutes, or until piping hot in the centre, following the instructions above.

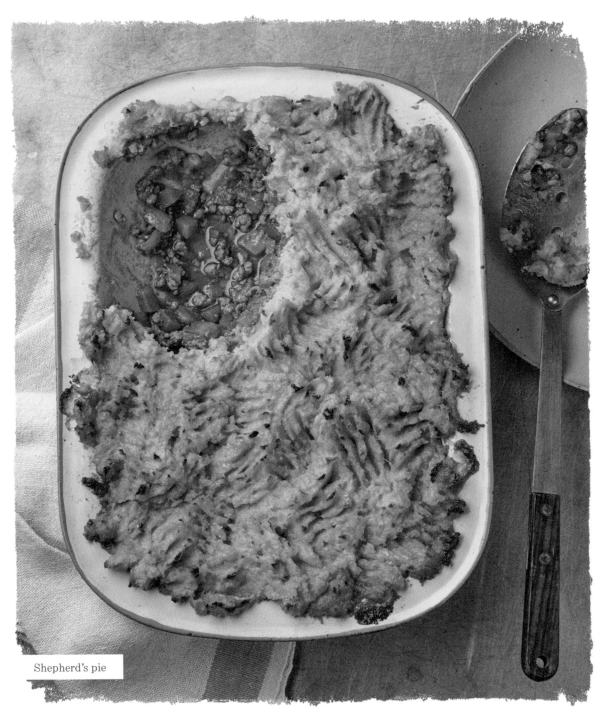

Shepherd's pie

SUCCESS
exercise plan

Phase Three is the final stage to a toned, firm, and fit body. It will take you approximately 45 minutes to complete. Over time you will be able to mix-and-match all the exercises from the 6 weeks to create your own plan. You will need a timer and two 2–3kg (4½–6½lb) dumbbells. You may also want a mat.

Work out with this exercise plan 3 or 4 days a week on the days of your choosing.

Do the indicated number of repetitions or hold time for each exercise. Complete a combo, take a 90 second rest, then repeat the combo twice more before moving onto the next combo.

Your warm up is the Squat, curl, and press (p174). Combos I–III are strength combos and Combo IV is a cardio combo.

Make sure that your posture is correct at all times, to avoid injuries and maximize results. Think about the movements you are performing and concentrate on the muscles that you are working and engaging.

Stay in the moment and focus on each movement to make your body work harder and get results quicker.

Remember to stay hydrated. Keep a water bottle close to your exercise mat and drink from it frequently during the short rest breaks. After working out, bear in mind that you will still need to top up with water regularly, to replace lost stocks and maximize the benefits for your muscles.

COMBO I

SQUAT, CURL, AND PRESS (p174)

Do 15 repetitions

TRICEPS DIPS (p176)

Do 15 repetitions

BICEPS CURLS (p178)

Do 15 repetitions

ELBOW PLANK HOLD (p180)

Hold for 60 seconds

Rest for 90 seconds

REPEAT COMBO I, INCLUDING REST, TWICE MORE

MOVE ON TO COMBO II

Weeks 5–6

COMPLETE COMBO I THREE TIMES · COMPLETE COMBO II THREE TIMES · COMPLETE COMBO III THREE TIMES · COMPLETE COMBO IV THREE TIMES · COMPLETE THE COOL DOWN

COMBO II	COMBO III	COMBO IV	COOL DOWN
SUMO SQUAT WITH BICEPS CURLS (p182) Do 15 repetitions	**REVERSE LUNGE AND SHOULDER PRESS** (p190) Do 15 repetitions each side	**JUMPING JACKS** (p198) Repeat for 20 seconds Rest for 10 seconds	**PEDALLING DOWNWARD DOG** (p210) Hold for 60 seconds
RUSSIAN TWIST (p184) Do 30 repetitions	**LYING CHEST FLY** (p192) Do 15 repetitions	**HIGH KNEES** (p200) Repeat for 20 seconds Rest for 10 seconds	**RUNNER'S LUNGE** (p212) Do for 60 seconds
PUSH UPS (p188) Do 15 repetitions	**V-SITS** (p194) Do 15 repetitions	**MOUNTAIN CLIMBERS** (p202) Repeat for 20 seconds Rest for 10 seconds	**CAT-COW** (p213) Do for 60 seconds
WALL SIT (p189) Hold for 60 seconds Rest for 90 seconds	**BENT-OVER ROW** (p196) Do 15 repetitions Rest for 90 seconds	**JUMPING LUNGES** (p204) Repeat for 20 seconds Rest for 10 seconds	
REPEAT COMBO II, INCLUDING REST, TWICE MORE	**REPEAT COMBO III, INCLUDING REST, TWICE MORE**	**JUMP SQUATS** (p206) Repeat for 20 seconds Rest for 10 seconds	
MOVE ON TO COMBO III	**MOVE ON TO COMBO IV**	**BURPEES** (p208) Repeat for 20 seconds Rest for 60 seconds	
		REPEAT COMBO IV, INCLUDING REST, TWICE MORE	
		MOVE ON TO THE COOL DOWN	

Squat, curl, and press

Remember to take your time with this exercise and make sure you break down the movement exactly as spelled out. When it comes to the upwards press, be sure not throw your arms – maintain control of your movements.

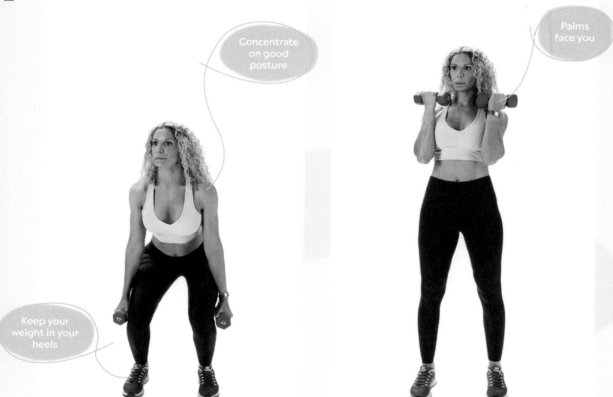

Concentrate on good posture

Palms face you

Keep your weight in your heels

1 Stand with your feet under your hips, holding a dumbbell in each hand with your arms by your sides. Bend your knees and lower your hips so your thighs are parallel to the floor.

2 Push through your heels to return to standing, while bringing the weights to your shoulders, performing a biceps curl.

WORK

Perform 15 repetitions.

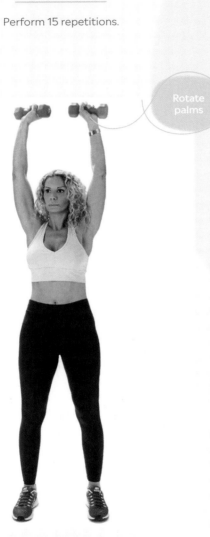

Rotate palms

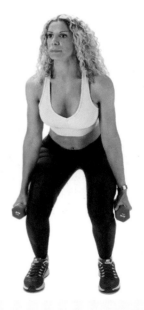

3 With your chest straight, keep your arms moving straight upwards, rotating your forearms so your palms face out.

4 Lower your arms back to your sides then return to the start position. This is one repetition. Perform 15 repetitions in total.

Triceps dips

Remember with this exercise that it's important to maintain good form. Make sure your elbows don't splay outwards when you dip down, and also be sure not to let your shoulders rise up or your head move.

WORK

Perform 15 repetitions.

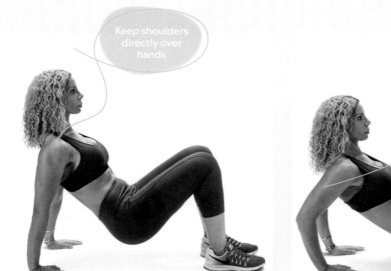

Keep shoulders directly over hands

Concentrate on using your triceps as opposed to your shoulders

1 Sit on the floor with your hands behind you, shoulder-width apart and fingers pointing forwards. Position your feet away from your bottom. Straighten your arms and lift your pelvis.

2 Keeping your pelvis high, inhale, then bend your elbows so they stick straight out behind you. Exhale while you straighten your arms. This completes one repetition. Do 15 repetitions.

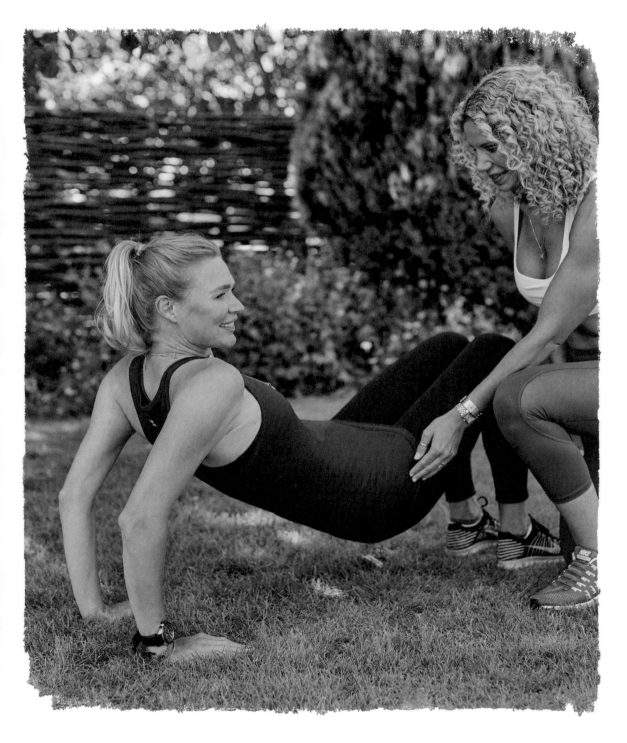

Biceps curls

When doing Biceps curls pay careful attention to the entire movement. When the dumbbells are down by your sides, make sure you bring them all the way back up close to your shoulders without curling your wrists. Always raise and lower them slowly and steadily while keeping your knees soft and your elbows in.

WORK

Perform 15 repetitions.

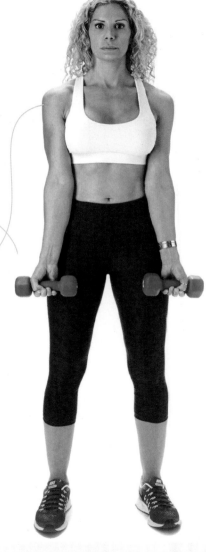

Concentrate on good posture

1 Stand tall with your knees soft. Hold a dumbbell in each hand, palms facing out, with your arms straight down and held close to your sides.

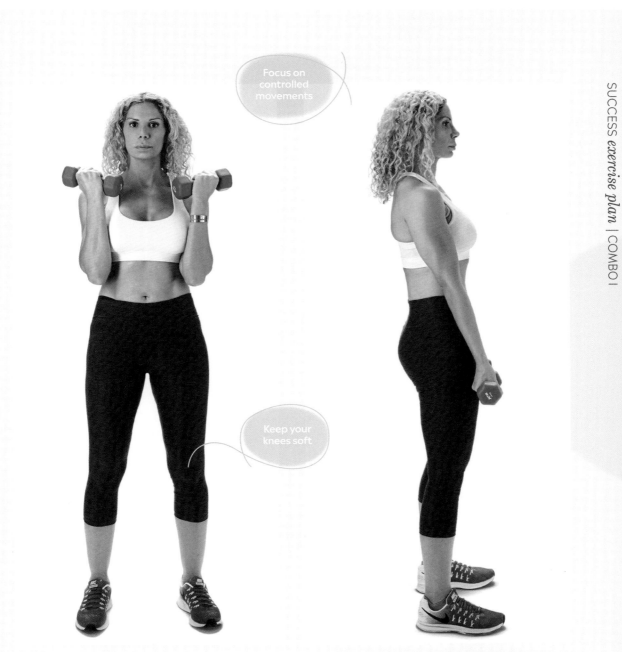

Focus on controlled movements

Keep your knees soft

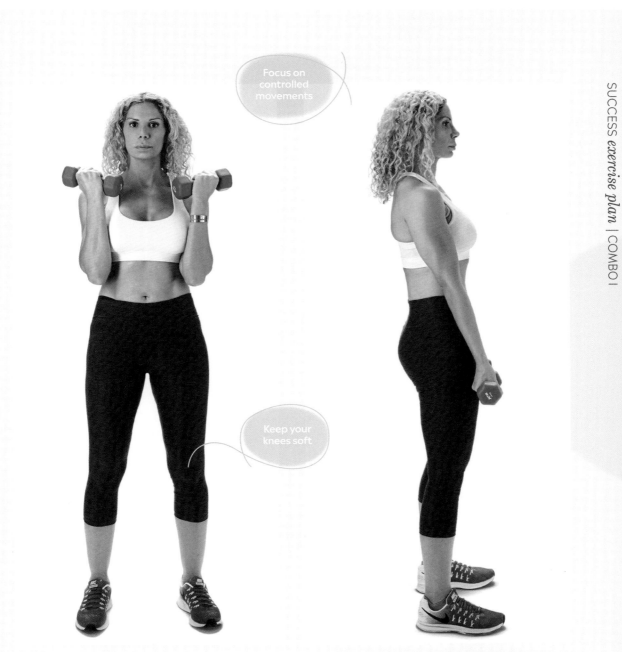

2 Keeping your elbows close to your sides, slowly raise both dumbbells to chest height. Be careful not to curl your wrists.

3 Slowly lower the dumbbells back to the starting position. This is one repetition. Do 15 repetitions.

Elbow plank hold

Alignment is everything here. Your elbows should be straight under your shoulders and your palms on the floor. Your body should be in one straight line from your head to your heels – don't let your hips dip or your bottom stick up.

WORK

Hold for 60 seconds.

Stack your elbows under your shoulders

Make sure your hips don't dip

1 Get down on the floor, resting on your forearms and knees.

"If you feel any pain in your shoulders, widen the gap between your feet."

- Amélie

Keep head aligned with spine

Engage your core to keep a straight back

2 Straighten your legs to lift your knees off the floor and shift your weight to your forearms and toes. Rest your weight mainly on your elbows.

3 Contract your core muscles to keep yourself up. Keep your back flat and don't let your bottom stick up. If your back droops, your core muscles are not working. Hold for 60 seconds.

Sumo squat with biceps curls

Unlike a normal squat, remember to keep your stance wide with your toes angled outwards. In order to really benefit from this exercise, be sure to focus on squeezing your bottom muscles as you push through your legs to stand back up.

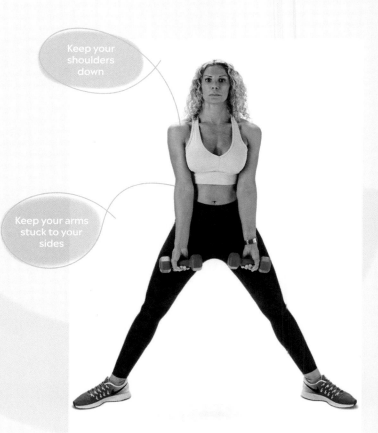

Keep your shoulders down

Keep your arms stuck to your sides

1 Hold a dumbbell in each hand, with your arms straight down in front of you and palms facing out. Place your heels just less that 1m (3ft) apart, with your toes pointing outwards.

WORK

Perform 15 repetitions.

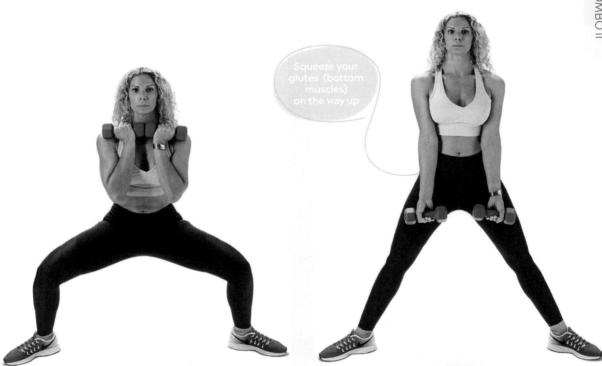

Squeeze your glutes (bottom muscles) on the way up

2 Keeping your weight in your heels and your shoulders over your hips, bend your knees to lower your hips. At the same time, bend your elbows to raise the dumbbells to shoulder height.

3 Straighten your legs and arms to return to the starting position. Squeeze the muscles in your bottom as you stand. This is one repetition. Perform a total of 15 repetitions.

Russian twist

For maximum effect when you're twisting side to side, keep your eyes on your hands. This way, both your gaze and your head follow your movements, increasing your upper-body stability.

WORK

Perform 30 repetitions.

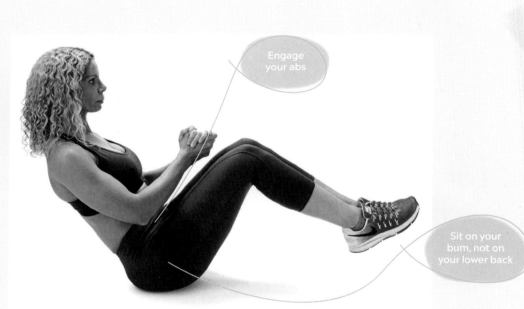

Engage your abs

Sit on your bum, not on your lower back

1 Sit on the ground with your knees bent. Pull your abs towards your spine, then lean back a few centimetres while lifting your feet off the floor. Be sure to keep your back straight. Clasp your hands in front of you with your elbows bent.

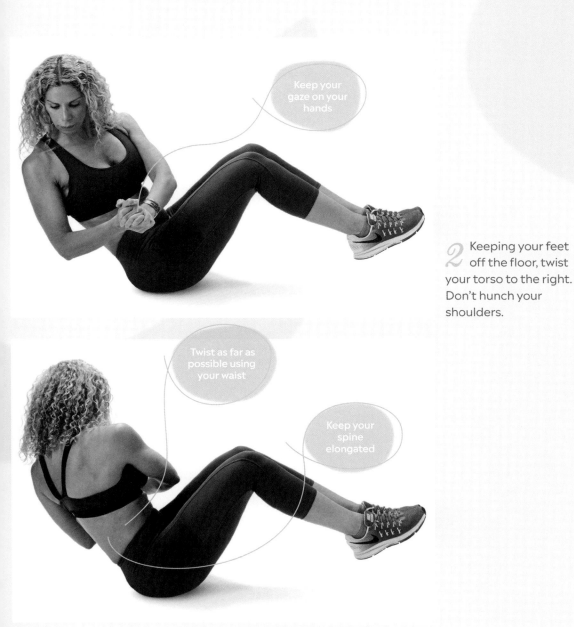

Keep your
gaze on your
hands

2 Keeping your feet
off the floor, twist
your torso to the right.
Don't hunch your
shoulders.

Twist as far as
possible using
your waist

Keep your
spine
elongated

3 Twist your torso to the left before
returning to centre. This is one repetition.
Perform 30 repetitions. To make it easier, you
can lower your heels to the ground if needed.

If I had a stressful day ahead and had done Amélie's exercises in the morning, I was more ready for the day's challenges. I felt calmer.

– Jodie

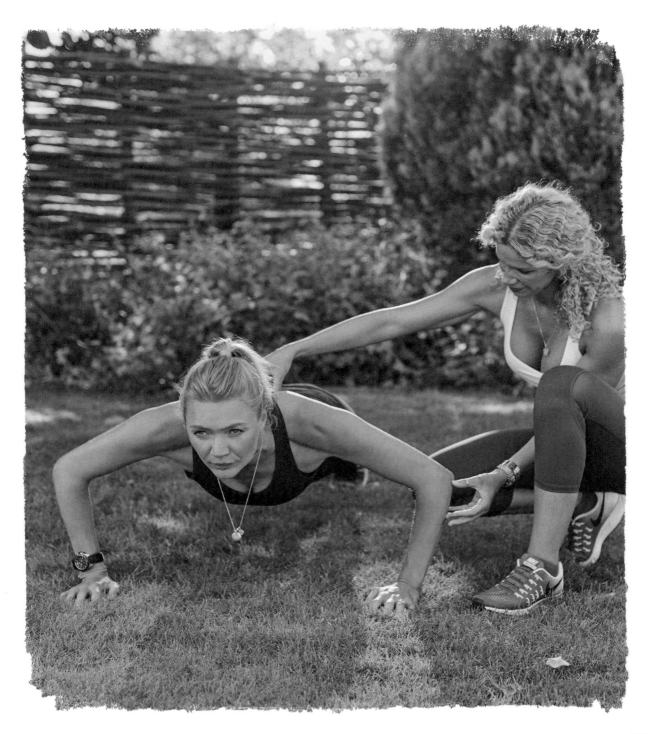

Push-ups

When doing a push-up, place your hands wide apart and make sure your shoulder blades don't touch as you go down. Pull your navel to your spine and engage your abdominal muscles. If you are struggling, position your feet 30cm (12in) apart for balance.

WORK

Perform 15 repetitions.

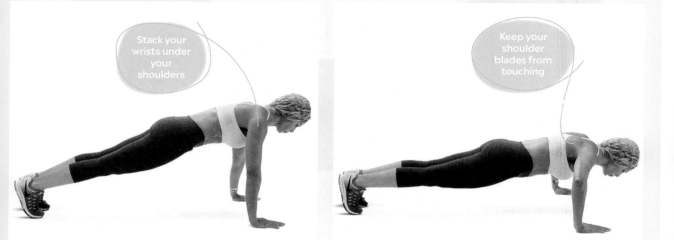

Stack your wrists under your shoulders

Keep your shoulder blades from touching

1 Begin in a High plank (see p64), with your body in a straight line. Pull your navel towards your spine. Don't let your hips drop or your lower back arch.

2 Bend your elbows out to the sides, lowering your body as you exhale. Pause at the bottom, then raise yourself back up to a High plank. This is one repetition. Perform a total of 15 repetitions.

Wall sit

This is a very simple exercise: the key is to keep your back totally flat on the wall. Pull your navel towards your spine, and take your time walking your feet away from the wall. When you feel pressure from knee-to-bottom, you've found the right distance. Don't slump, and don't let your knees rise higher than your waist.

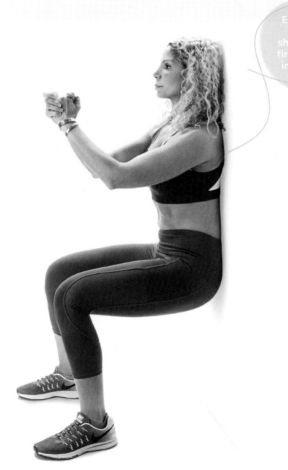

Ensure your back and shoulders are firmly pushed into the wall

WORK

Hold for 60 seconds.

1 Stand with your back pressing against a wall.

2 Slide downwards into a squat position by walking your feet forwards until your knees make a right angle and your thighs are parallel to the floor. Hold for 60 seconds.

Reverse lunge and shoulder press

Remember to make sure your actions are controlled during this movement. Keep your core muscles engaged at all times to help achieve this.

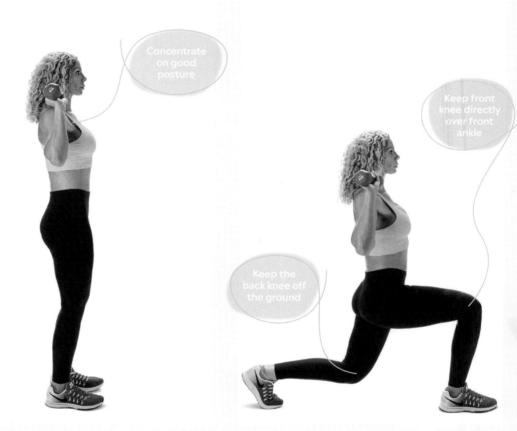

Concentrate on good posture

Keep front knee directly over front ankle

Keep the back knee off the ground

1 Stand tall with your feet together. Hold the dumbbells at shoulder height, with your palms facing slightly upwards.

2 Step your left foot back to drop into a lunge, bending both knees at right angles. The back knee should point towards the ground. Focus on achieving depth, not length.

WORK

Perform 15 repetitions
on each side, alternating.

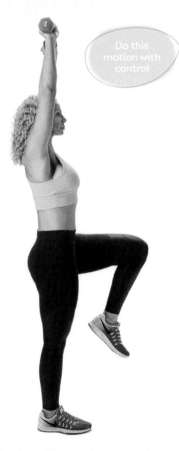

Do this motion with control

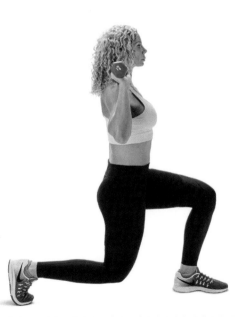

3 Pushing off with your left foot, drive your left knee up and forwards until it is at the same height as your waist. At the same time, raise your arms straight above your head.

4 Return to the starting position. This is one repetition. To repeat, step back into a lunge again, this time with your right foot behind you. Perform 15 repetitions on each side, alternating.

191

Lying chest fly

With this exercise remember to consciously push your back and feet into the floor. Don't let your hands touch down at the bottom of the movement, but keep them about 5cm (2in) off the ground. That way you can be sure your chest muscles are really working.

WORK

Perform 15 repetitions.

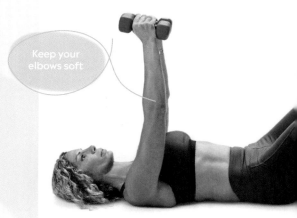

Relax your neck muscles

Keep your elbows soft

1 Holding a dumbbell in each hand, lie on your back with your hips and knees both bent and your feet flat on the ground. Press your lower back into the ground.

2 Raise your arms towards the ceiling, palms facing each other, keeping the elbows slig bent and making sure the weights do not touc

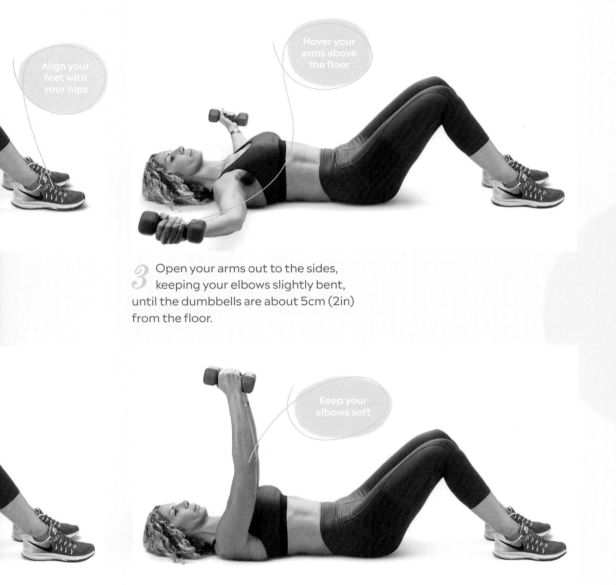

Align your
feet with
your hips

Hover your
arms above
the floor

3 Open your arms out to the sides,
keeping your elbows slightly bent,
until the dumbbells are about 5cm (2in)
from the floor.

Keep your
elbows soft

4 Raise your arms back towards the ceiling, bringing
the weights together over your chest without
them touching. This is one repetition. Repeat Steps 2–4
for a total of 15 repetitions.

V-sits

Your spine should be in a straight line, as though you have a thread pulling you straight from the coccyx to the base of your head. Do not hunch your shoulders, use your neck at all, or tuck your chin into your chest. Manage your abilities and choose the right position for you – don't be too ambitious to start with. If you feel your back hurting, change your position until your abs are working instead.

WORK

Perform 15 repetitions.

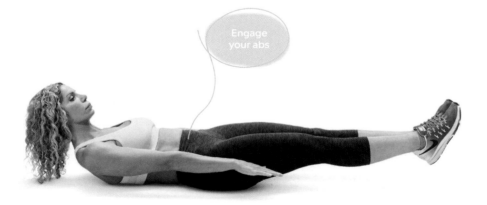

Engage your abs

1 Lie on your back with your hands by your sides, then raise your arms off the floor. Engage your abs and lift your legs until they are raised off the floor.

"If you feel pain in your lower back, don't lean back as far when doing the crunch movement."

— Amélie

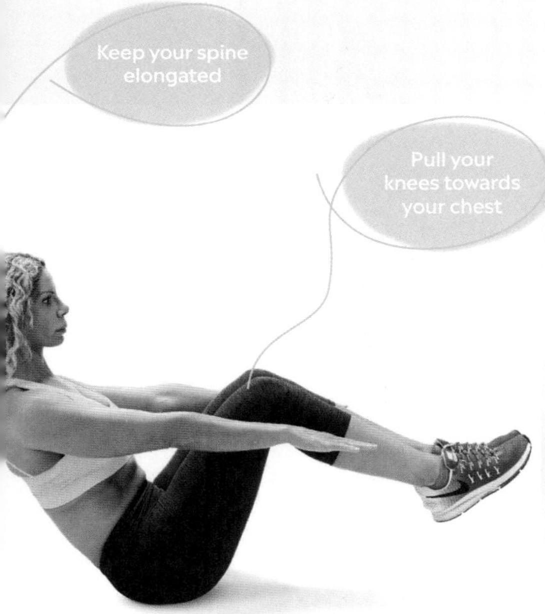

Keep your spine elongated

Pull your knees towards your chest

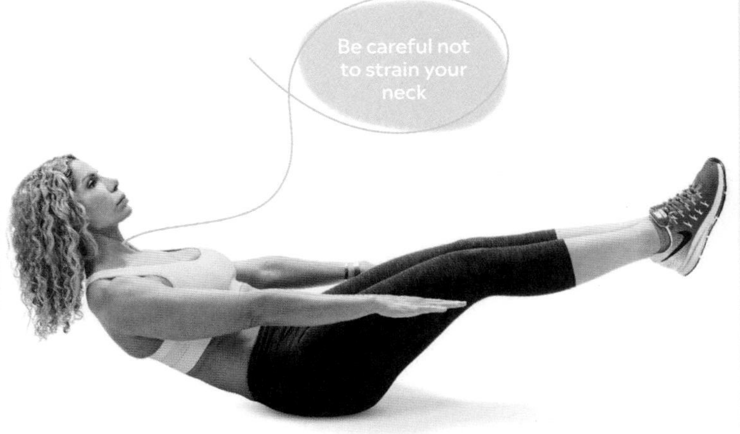

Be careful not to strain your neck

2 Use your abs to lift your head and torso off the floor, and bend your knees. Make sure the pressure of this movement is resting on your lower abs and not in your lower back.

3 Slowly lower your torso and straighten your legs until your back is on the floor, but your head, shoulders, arms, and legs are raised. This is one repetition. Repeat Steps 2 and 3 for 15 repetitions.

Bent-over row

Remember that for this exercise you need soft knees and a straight back. Keep your arms and elbows by your sides, squeeze your shoulder blades together, and release the weights down slowly.

WORK

Perform 15 repetitions.

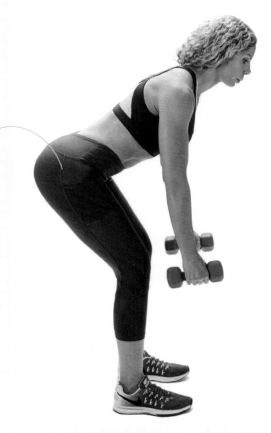

Lean forwards from the hips

1 Holding a dumbbell in each hand, extend your arms so they are straight. Lean forwards with a straight back. Keep your knees soft and pull your navel towards your spine.

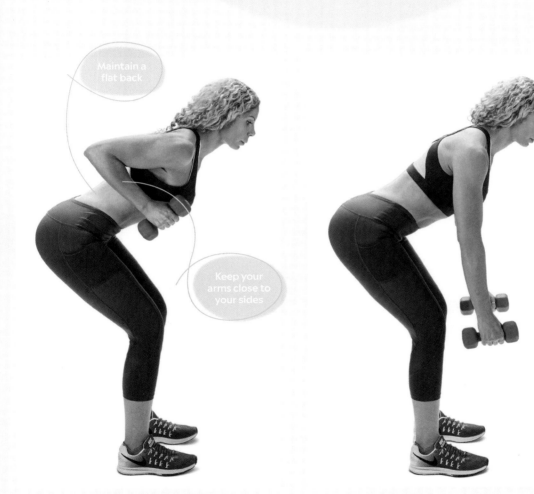

2 Lift the dumbbells straight up to chest level by bending your elbows up behind you, squeezing your shoulder blades together. Keep your elbows in and pointed upwards.

3 Slowly lower the weights back to the starting position. This is one repetition. Repeat Steps 2 and 3 for a total of 15 repetitions.

COMBO IV

This is the cardio segment of the workout. Do each exercise for 20 seconds, take a 10-second rest, and progress to the next exercise. Take a 60-second break, then repeat Combo IV twice more, to make a total of three sets.

Jumping jacks

Now that you've mastered this exercise from Phase One, try to add a little more speed. Remember that you must maintain control of your limbs though, or you will not benefit from the movement. Keep the muscles in your arms, legs, and core engaged, and concentrate on your posture throughout.

WORK

Repeat the exercise for 20 seconds, then take a 10-second rest.

Concentrate on good posture

1 Stand tall with your feet together and your arms by your sides. Keep your knees soft and make sure your posture is good, with your navel drawn towards your spine.

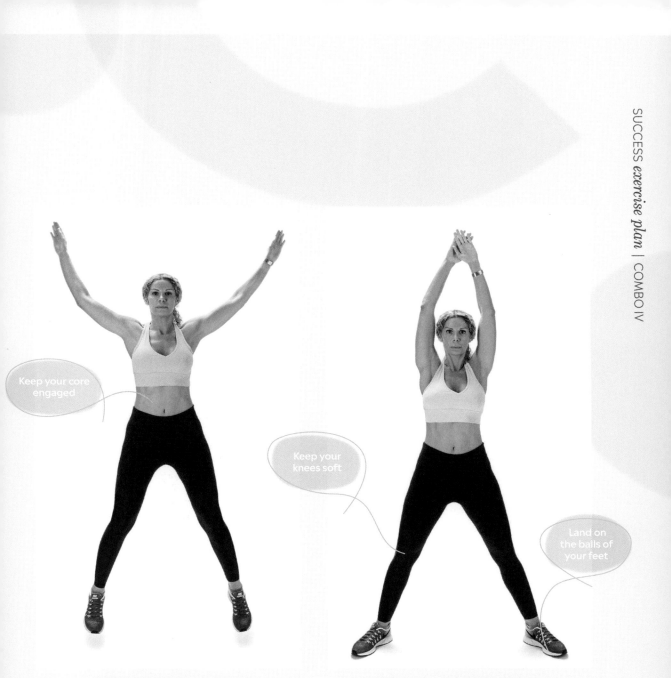

Keep your core engaged

Keep your knees soft

Land on the balls of your feet

2 Jump off the balls of your feet as you spread out your arms and legs to a wide star position. While your jump should be energetic, it should also be controlled.

3 Land with your feet apart and your hands touching over your head. Jump again, returning through the wide star position before landing with your feet together and your arms by your sides, as in Step 1. Repeat for 20 seconds.

High knees

With this exercise remember that you're not trying to sprint in place, you're trying to raise your knees up to belly button height. Be sure to stay on the balls of your feet, keep your core engaged, and don't hunch. Move your knees towards your torso, not your torso towards your knees.

WORK

Repeat the exercise for 20 seconds, then take a 10-second rest.

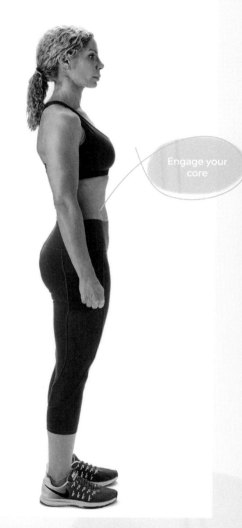

Engage your core

1 Stand tall with your feet together.

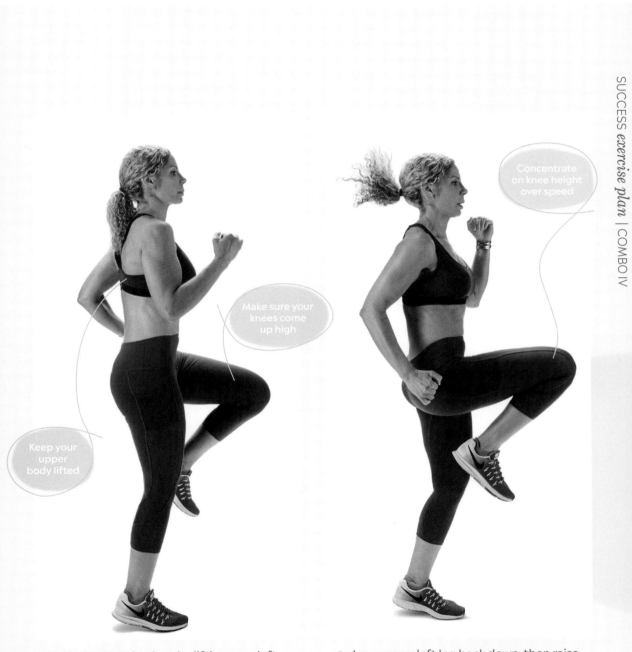

2 Begin to run in place by lifting your left knee high in front of you to the level of your waist. Engage your core as the knee comes up. Pump your arms at the same time.

3 Lower your left leg back down, then raise your right knee, swinging your arms in the opposite direction. Repeat for 20 seconds.

Mountain climbers

Now that you're familiar with this exercise from Phase One, try to add a little more speed – without losing your form – in order to get the cardiovascular benefits. Remember, it's like low-impact sprinting. Mountain climbers will work your abs, triceps, shoulders, and core muscles.

WORK

Repeat the exercise for 20 seconds, then take a 10-second rest.

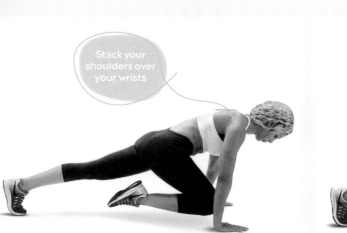

Stack your shoulders over your wrists

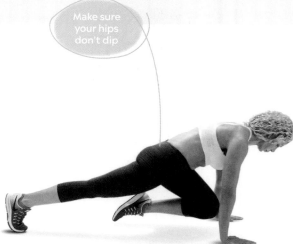

Make sure your hips don't dip

1 Start in a High plank (see p64). Bring your right knee to your chest, shifting your weight into your hands.

2 Switch legs quickly, bringing the left knee forwards while moving the right foot back. Repeat for 20 seconds. Your feet should barely touch the floor as they swap back and forth, as if running.

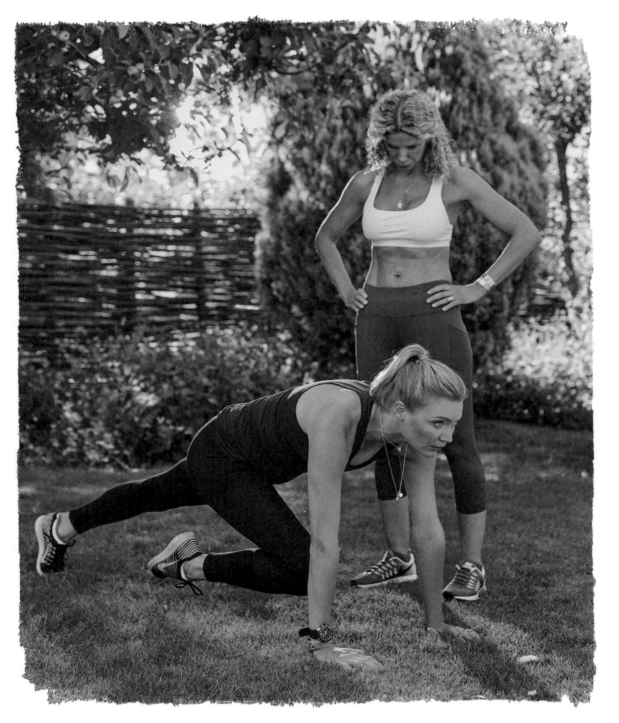

Jumping lunges

This exercise is designed to get your heart rate up! The key is to lunge both far and fast. It's a fairly low-impact exercise. Make sure your back stays straight, and use your arms as "propellers" to power the movement.

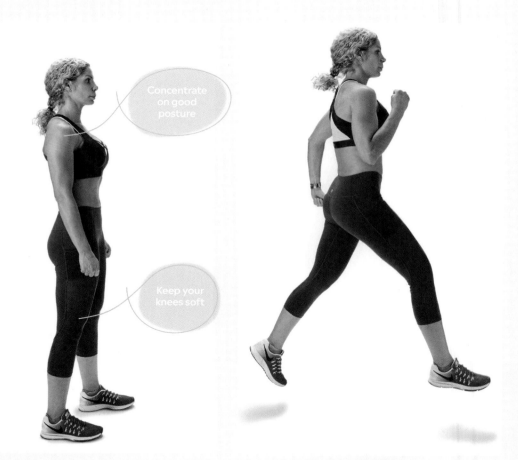

Concentrate on good posture

Keep your knees soft

1 Stand tall with your left foot slightly in front of your right. Make sure you're not too stiff; keep your stance active with your knees soft.

2 With your core engaged, push off with both feet into a jump. Switch the position of your feet in mid-air so your right leg comes forwards and your left leg goes back.

WORK

Repeat the exercise for
20 seconds, then take a
10-second rest.

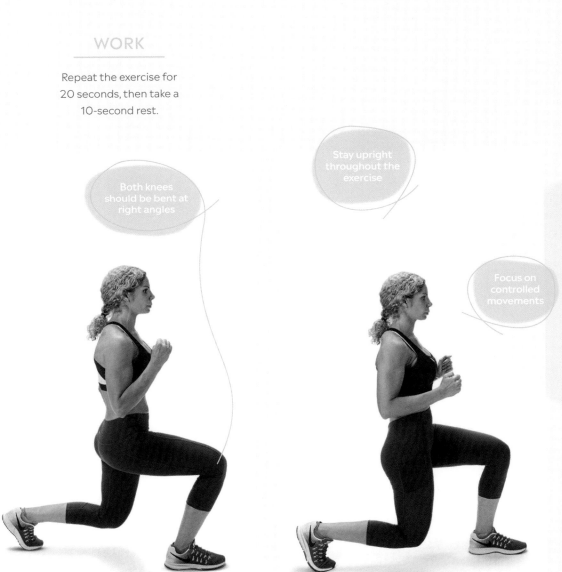

Both knees
should be bent at
right angles

Stay upright
throughout the
exercise

Focus on
controlled
movements

3 Land in a lunge with your right leg in front. The back knee should point towards the floor; the front knee should be no further forwards than your toes.

4 Immediately push off again and switch legs in mid-air once more. Without rest, repeat this movement, alternating which leg is in front. Repeat for 20 seconds.

Jump squats

Remember that Jump squats are an explosive movement – use your arms to propel the jump. As with any squat, use your core to keep you stable. To protect your knees, try to land on your full foot, not just your toes.

WORK

Repeat the exercise for 20 seconds, then take a 10-second rest.

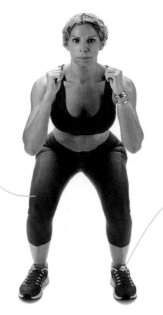

Keep knees behind toes

Keep weight in heels

1 Stand with your feet hip-width apart, with your arms by your sides. Bend your knees, lowering your hips so your thighs are parallel to the floor.

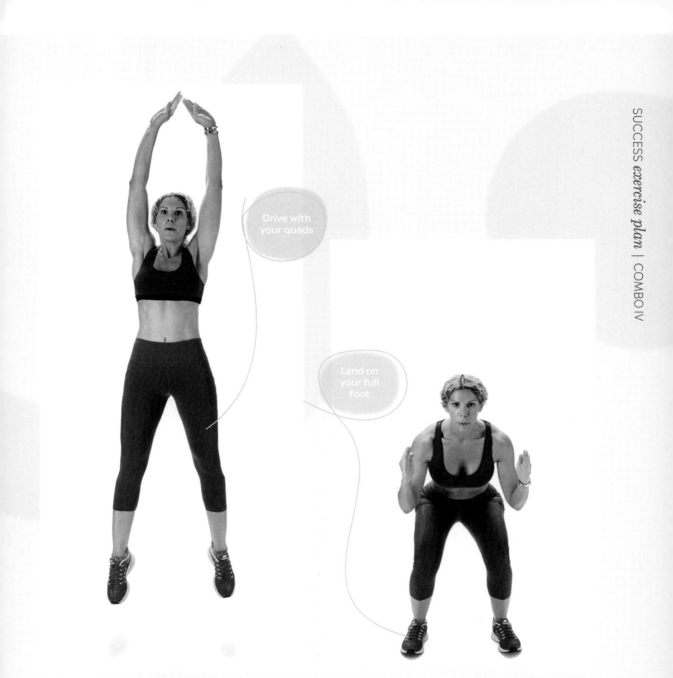

Drive with your quads

Land on your full foot

2 Swing your arms to the ceiling as you jump straight up, pushing off with both feet.

3 Land softly on your full feet, not your toes, as you return to the squat position. Repeat for 20 seconds.

PHASE THREE *weeks 5–6*

Burpees

Remember that the key to doing the super-technical burpee is to control your movements at all times by using your core. After the High plank, be sure to jump your feet back in to propel yourself up in to the jump – you should aim to have your knees at chest level, not behind you, before you jump. Also, keep your movements smooth so that you don't hurt yourself.

WORK

Repeat the exercise for 20 seconds, then take a 60-second rest.

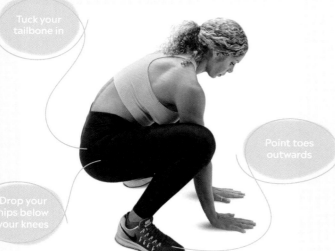

Tuck your tailbone in

Keep your legs straight

Point toes outwards

Drop your hips below your knees

1 Stand with your feet wider than hip-width apart. Push your hips back, and bend your knees to come into a low, wide squat. Place your hands on the floor.

2 Do a squat thrust by jumping your feet back into a High plank (see p64) position; your hands should be under your shoulders and your feet hip-width apart.

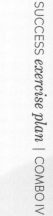

3 Slowly lower your chest to the floor by bending your elbows outwards, then straighten them and press up to lift your body back into a High plank.

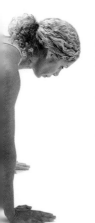

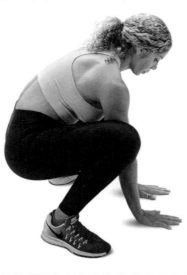

Drive off the toes

4 Jump your feet towards your hands, coming back into a squat. Really jump your feet in to give momentum for the next step.

5 Do an explosive jump straight up, getting as much height as you can, to complete one burpee. Repeat for 20 seconds.

COOL DOWN

Your cool down should take three minutes: do each of these stretches for 60 seconds.

Pedalling down dog

The key to Pedalling down dog is to really go up on to your tiptoes to feel the stretch from ankle to glute. Make sure, when you reset, that your entire foot is on the floor.

WORK

Perform this stretch for 60 seconds.

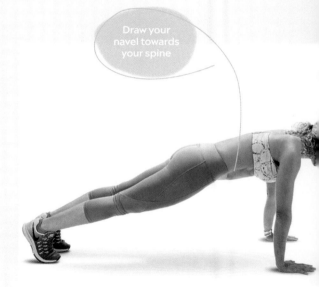

Draw your navel towards your spine

1 Begin in a High plank (see p64) with your body in a straight line, hands under your shoulders, and feet hip-width apart. Don't let your hips drop or your lower back arch.

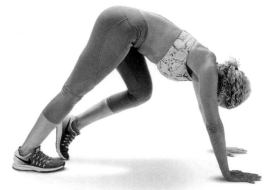

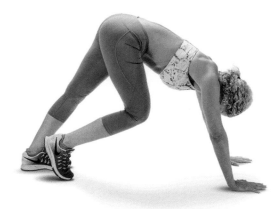

2 Lift your pelvis up and back, making a v-shape with your body. (Walk your feet towards your hands if you need to.) Start "pedalling" by pressing down on one heel while bending the other leg.

3 Hold for a few seconds, then switch legs. Lightly pedal back and forth for 60 seconds.

211

Runner's lunge

Having learned this stretch in Phase One, you should be more comfortable with going a little deeper into the lunge this time. Really feel the stretch, but remember to go gently.

WORK

Perform this stretch for 60 seconds.

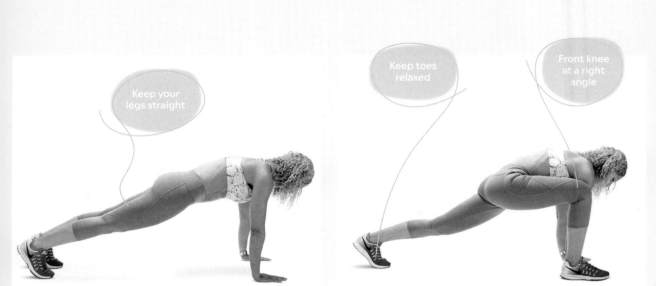

Keep your legs straight

Keep toes relaxed

Front knee at a right angle

1 Start in a High plank (see p64) with your hands directly under your shoulders and your body in one straight line.

2 Step your right foot forwards so it sits to the outside of your hands. Hold briefly, then repeat on your left side. Continue to swap back and forth from side to side for a total of 60 seconds.

Cat-cow

Cat-cow is a mind and body stretch. Your breathing is everything. Slowly inhale, pushing your neck back, then exhale as you tuck your chin into your chest and round your back to the point where your shoulder blades come apart. Don't rush it!

WORK

Perform this stretch for 60 seconds.

Spread your shoulder blades wide

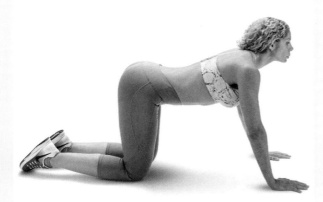

1 Get on your hands and knees, with your knees under your hips and your wrists under your shoulders. Begin in a neutral spine position, with your back flat and your abs engaged. As you inhale, let your belly soften, arch your back, and lift your head and tailbone. This part of the stretch is called "Cow".

2 As you exhale, round your spine up to the ceiling, pulling your navel towards your spine and simultaneously tucking in your tailbone and chin. This part of the stretch is called "Cat". Continue flowing back and forth from Cat to Cow, breathing deeply so as not to rush each movement.

213

Jodie & Amélie's
FINAL WRAP-UP

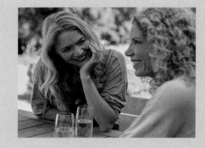

Amélie
You've finished! How did you find it overall?

Jodie
It was difficult in the beginning, but then your body starts to thank you. I was always aware of the benefits and importance of having a healthy body, but your programme takes you to another level of feeling brilliant, strong, clear-headed, and more aware.

Amélie
Would you say you had an Achilles' heel?

Amélie
Have you felt your fitness improve?

Jodie
I can manage the physical side of things just fine. The mental side is usually my downfall. My inner voice sometimes undermines me and tells me I won't succeed. Your plan has helped me to reset my brain.

Jodie
Yes, the workouts got easier as my body adapted, but I need to put in the effort and set aside the time. The thing is, none of your exercises is hideous. I feel every part of my body is being worked, so I want to do them again.

"

Amélie

How did you fit in the exercise if you had a massively busy day?

Jodie

My life has always been physically active. If I knew I was going to have a really busy day where I would be on my feet in the pub, then I would take a view. I'd make an educated guess at the beginning of the day as to whether or not I needed to fit in your exercises in the morning.

Amélie

How was the food plan?

Jodie

Great – I have more energy and mental clarity, and I'm definitely more aware of the pleasures of eating and the flavours of food. I savour every mouthful. My body feels cleared out and the food keeps me full. I've found new, lovely ways of using food. I used to look at pulses and grains and think "I know they're good for me, but they just taste so boring." Now I've got loads of ideas from using your recipes.

Amélie

Have your learned anything else about food?

Amélie

Have you noticed any other changes or improvements in your general health?

Jodie

That portion control is important. I needed to learn what the correct amount of food looked like on my plate. I also learned that it's important to sit down to eat, and to be conscious of the food while you're eating.

Jodie

Yes, the workouts made me feel relaxed and as though I could take on the world. I'm sleeping better. I'm not awake at 4 or 5 in the morning. Getting a full night's sleep makes me calmer, and I feel like I'm making better decisions. Not putting all those stimulants from unhealthy food into my body must be helping with that, too.

"

Balance your life
THE WAY FORWARD

Congratulations! Now that you've finished the six-week plan your mind and body should feel in excellent shape. You will want to stay that way, and I want to help you do that. Here are some of the things to remember to stay balanced and healthy in mind and body forever. Stick to your new habits and they will serve you well for life.

Food

1 **Always remain in charge** and aware of what you put into your mouth. Remember, if it's not water, it's food. It doesn't matter if you ate it standing up or walking or, worst of all, you didn't notice eating it and forgot about it straight away. You still ate it.

2 **Have three meals a day.** If you're not a breakfast person, eat a little bit later. Try not to go without food until lunchtime because it has a knock-on effect and you will be ravenous by 9pm. And by then, when you're tired and trying to relax, your discipline will go out the window.

3 **Eat a lot of vegetables**, a little less protein, and even less carbohydrates. Stick to wholegrain bread, rice, and pasta, and eat sweet potatoes rather than regular potatoes. That's as basic as it gets. Make room for fruit, but in a balanced way: it's not okay to go through a whole punnet of grapes in one sitting.

4 **Never eat anything straight out of the packaging.** Instead, transfer the correct serving size to a plate so you can control your portions.

5 Portion control is not only about putting **the right amount of food** on your plate at every mealtime, it's also about balance. If you had a big breakfast, have a small lunch. If you had a week of indulging, have a fortnight of watching what you eat and maybe go back to Phase One of my plan (see pp18–81).

6 Watching what you eat is not a punishment and eating is not just about putting fuel in your body. **Enjoy your food.** Sit down to eat it. Treat every meal as a mini event!

7 Walk away from the notion that you deserve a "treat" when it comes to food. Food is not a security blanket. It won't fix feelings. The same applies to alcohol. Let's all try to **be less emotional about what we eat and drink**.

Exercise

1 **Training is the best way** to be clear-headed and happy. It makes you strong and empowers you in many different ways, strengthening you both physically and mentally. Training also gives your mind a break when you need it, and is a very satisfying thing to do. When you start seeing the results, you find yourself at the centre of a virtuous circle: you'll realize you don't want to ruin your efforts, so you will also try harder to eat well.

2 It's a trope, but it's true: **you cannot out-train a bad diet.** Forget the idea that because you worked out in the morning you can indulge later in the day. That will cancel out all the benefits of the training.

3 Whatever exercise you're doing, **keep doing it.** Adapt it to achieve the results you want. Micro training (focusing on one specific area) may be frowned upon, but if there is a part of your training that you feel needs more attention, it's okay to concentrate on it.

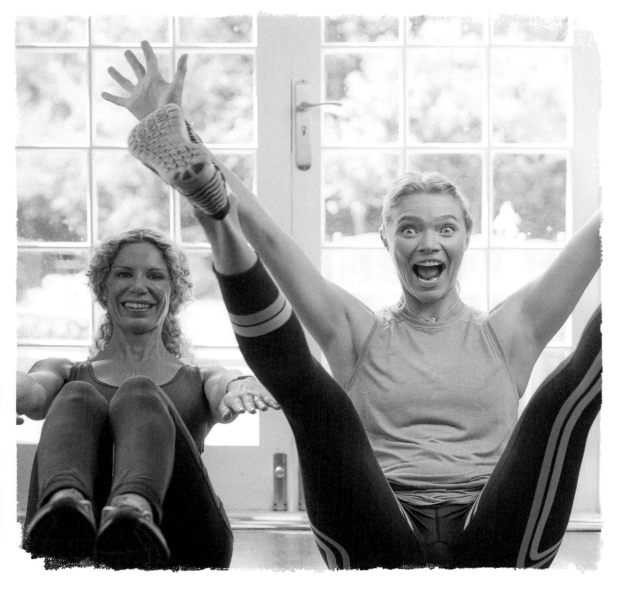

4 **Keep it fun and keep it varied**. If you feel your motivation waning, try to recruit a friend, or find a club to encourage you tc keep going. Whether it's to be slimmer or healthier, don't lose sight of why you started the programme in the first place.

5 Remember that you cannot go wrong by **looking after yourself**. It's one of the few things you can indulge in with no downside.

Index

About the authors

JODIE KIDD

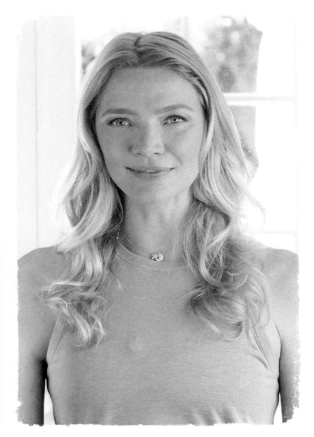

Jodie Kidd is best known for being a television presenter and one of the most successful models of her generation.

Having been discovered at the age of just 15, she shot into the spotlight, appeared on the cover of *Vogue*, opened shows for Givenchy, and walked for Alexander McQueen's debut runway presentation. She travelled the world as an international model, then returned to the catwalk in 2013 to walk for Moschino during Milan Fashion Week, and the following year was the face of Jaeger's Autumn Winter campaign.

Jodie has enjoyed a successful career as a high-octane Maserati racing driver, competing at some of Europe's most prestigious racing circuits and racing for Jaguar in the legendary Mille Miglia. She has also taken on many endurance challenges including L'Etape du Tour and, after becoming an ambassador for the charity Help for Heroes, Jodie completed the Burma Bike Ride, the Big Battlefield Bike Ride, and climbed Mount Kilimanjaro to raise money on their behalf.

She has taken part in several popular television programmes, including BBC One's *Who Do You Think You Are* and *Strictly Come Dancing*. She also presented her own US television show *Fashion Avenue*, and her own BBC Three documentary *I Believe in Miracle Healing*, and has co-presented Channel 5's *The Classic Car Show* and ITV's coverage of The Isle of Man TT.

Jodie is passionate about sustainability and growing her own vegetables and is a keen cook, having been a finalist in *Celebrity MasterChef*. In 2017, Jodie opened gastropub The Half Moon in Kirdford and the following year it was awarded 2 Rosettes by the AA. Jodie is involved in menu design and the creation of dishes, as well as hosting her very own curry night each month. Guests can expect flavour and quality to be at the centre of everything with British produce enhanced by global flavours inspired by Jodie's travels.

Jodie enjoys living in the countryside with her son, Indio.

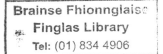
221

About the authors

AMÉLIE KHELLAF-GOVETT

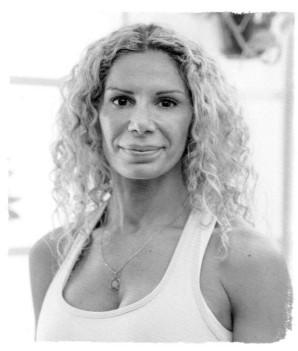

Paris-born Amélie Khellaf-Govett enjoyed a successful international career in PR and Marketing before choosing London as her base. Her passion for wellness led her to retrain as a Personal Trainer and Nutritionist.

By developing her own training and eating programmes, Amélie supports her clients in achieving their goals, maintaining new standards, and feeling confident in their abilities.

It is through taking a personal approach with every client that Amélie successfully shares her balanced approach to fitness and nutrition.

Amélie was voted one of *Tatler*'s top 5 personal trainers in 2016 and 2017 and *Cosmo* quoted her as "The go-to personal trainer behind some of London's most powerful business women".

Acknowledgments

DK would like to thank the following people for their contributions to the book:

Food stylist **Jane Lawrie**
Hair and make-up **Susana Mota**
Indexer **Marie Lorimer**
Photographers **William Reavell and Rob Streeter**
Prop stylist **Rob Merrett**
Recipe tester for Jodie's recipes **Jane Lawrie**

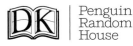

Senior Editor Kathryn Meeker
Project Art Editor Harriet Yeomans
Editors Lucy Bannell, Claire Cross, Toby, Mann,
and Constance Novis
Designers Tessa Bindloss, Louise Brigenshaw,
and Glenda Fisher
Editorial Assistant Poppy Blakiston-Houston
Jacket Designer Nicola Powling
Image Post Production Adam Brackenbury, Sunil Sharma,
Rajdeep Singh, Neeraj Bhatia, and Pankaj Sharma
Jackets Coordinator Lucy Philpott
Senior Producer, Pre-Production Tony Phipps
Senior Producer Stephanie McConnell
Managing Editor Stephanie Farrow
Managing Art Editor Christine Keilty
Art Director Maxine Pedliham
Publishing Director Mary-Clare Jerram

First published in Great Britain in 2019
by Dorling Kindersley Limited
80 Strand, London, WC2R 0RL

A CIP catalogue record for this book
is available from the British Library.
ISBN: 978-0-2413-6414-7

Printed and bound in China.

A WORLD OF IDEAS:
SEE ALL THERE IS TO KNOW
www.dk.com

"And Amélie says it's fine to have the odd glass of wine."

- Jodie